DOCUMENTATION PLANNING FOR THE U.S. HEALTH CARE SYSTEM

DOCUMENTATION PLANNING FOR THE U.S. HEALTH CARE SYSTEM

Edited by

JOAN D. KRIZACK

née HAAS

THE JOHNS HOPKINS UNIVERSITY PRESS

Baltimore and London

For Rebekah (who's always first in my book),
Nanny, Dapes, Carol, Barbara, Marc, and Rocky.

© 1994 The Johns Hopkins University Press
All rights reserved
Printed in the United States of America on acid-free paper

The Johns Hopkins University Press
2715 North Charles Street
Baltimore, Maryland 21218-4319
The Johns Hopkins Press Ltd., London

Library of Congress Cataloging-in-Publication Data

Documentation planning for the U.S. health care system / edited by Joan D. Krizack.
     p.   cm.
   Includes bibliographical references and index.
   ISBN 0-8018-4805-9 (acid-free paper)
   1. Archives, Medical—United States.   2. Medical records—Management—United
States.   I. Krizack, Joan D.
   R119.8.D63   1994
   651.5'04261'0973—dc20   94-9566
                                                                   CIP

A catalog record for this book is available from the British Library.

CONTENTS

CHAPTER 5

CHAPTER 6

CHAPTER 7

CHAPTER 8

APPENDIX A

APPENDIX B

LIST OF CONTRIBUTORS

Paul G. Anderson, Ph.D., Associate Director for Archives and the History of Medicine, Washington University School of Medicine, St. Louis, Missouri

James G. Carson, Ph.D., Independent Archival Consultant, Chicago, Illinois, and former Curator of the American Medical Association Historical Health Fraud Alternative Medicine Collection

Peter B. Hirtle, M.A., M.L.S., Archives Specialist, Technology Research Staff, National Archives and Records Administration, Washington, D.C.

James J. Kopp, Ph.D., Vice President, Library Systems, P.S.S., Ltd., Reston, Virginia

Joan D. Krizack, M.A.T., M.S., Hospital Archivist, Children's Hospital, Boston, Massachusetts

Nancy McCall, M.L.A., Archivist, the Alan Mason Chesney Medical Archives, the Johns Hopkins Medical Institutions, Baltimore, Maryland

Lisa A. Mix, M.L.A., Processing Coordinator, The Alan Mason Chesney Medical Archives, the Johns Hopkins Medical Institutions, Baltimore, Maryland

ACKNOWLEDGMENTS

My first debts of gratitude are to the National Historical Publications and Records Commission, which funded this project, and to the Andrew J. Mellon Foundation, the Research Division of the National Endowment for the Humanities, and the University of Michigan for funding earlier research on hospitals. A special thanks is due to André Mayer for his insightful criticism and unflagging support throughout. I also wish to thank fellow archivists who offered advice and encouragement: Frank Boles, Megan Sniffin-Marinoff, David W. Nathan, Jeffrey L. Storchio, Joan Warnow-Blewett, and Nancy W. Zinn. Thanks to Helen W. Samuels and the Mellon group: Bruce H. Breummer, Bridget Carr, Terry Cook, James M. O'Toole, and D. Gregory Sanford, for stimulating discussions of functional analysis which resulted in refinements of this work. Co-conspirators Paul G. Anderson, James G. Carson, Peter B. Hirtle, James J. Kopp, Nancy McCall, and Lisa A. Mix deserve thanks and congratulations for enduring my seemingly endless requests for revisions. Several Johns Hopkins University faculty and staff members offered valuable criticism: Karen Butter, Elizabeth Fee, Alan Lyles, Harry Marks, and Robert Miller. I also wish to thank Wallace Daly for unlocking the mysteries of RLIN and Peter Carini for providing eleventh-hour reference service. Finally, I am indebted to Anne Malone and Peggy Slasman for allowing me to refine the documentation planning process at Children's Hospital and to the rest of the staff of the Development and Public Affairs Office for their computer expertise, friendship, and support.

INTRODUCTION

JOAN D. KRIZACK

During the 1970s, the archival profession began to question the methods it used to select records for preservation. In a series of seminal articles, F. Gerald Ham challenged archivists to rethink their traditional approach to appraisal and devise a methodology suited to selecting modern records produced by modern institutions.[1] Several archivists accepted Ham's challenge and wrote books grounded in the assumption that appraisal is based on disciplinary or institutional functions and activities.[2] For reasons that are not apparent, this approach to appraisal first took hold in the fields of science and technology, but by the mid-1980s archivists began to translate the new methodology to other fields.[3]

All of this work was based on the belief that archivists need to understand the context in which records are created (i.e., the functions and activities that generate records) before they can make appropriate appraisal decisions. The principle that appraisal must be grounded in an understanding of context had been advocated at least since the mid-1950s,[4] but it had not previously been incorporated into selection methodologies.

The focus of appraisal research shifted from disciplines to institutions after Helen Willa Samuels introduced the "documentation strategy" concept in 1985.[5] As defined by Patricia Aronsson, Larry Hackman, and Samuels, a documentation strategy is an interinstitutional approach to documenting an "ongoing issue, activity, or geographic area."[6] Samuels's article and the documentation strategy concept reinforced the notion that analysis and planning are necessary first steps in the appraisal or selection process. Samuels also assumed the absolute necessity of an active approach to selecting documentation, something that Howard Zinn, Hans Booms, F. Gerald Ham, and others had begun advocating in the 1970s.[7]

The archival community had mixed reactions to the concept of documentation strategy, which was often interpreted in ways other than had been intended; nonetheless, several archivists boldly attempted to apply the concept. The proposed documentation strategy for the high-technology companies located around Route 128 in Massachusetts by Alexander and Samuels never advanced beyond the hypothetical level,[8] and Cox's actual but unfinished attempt to carry out a documentation strategy for western New York raised substantive issues about the concept's practicality and viability.[9] Two retrospective applications of the documentation strategy concept—one to analyze the range of topics of collections already held by manuscript repositories and the other applied to a historical topic, nineteenth-century quartz mining in Northern California—were more successful.[10]

In conducting research on the U.S. health care system and thinking about how to apply the documentation strategy concept to health care in Massachusetts, I came to the conclusion that the theory underlying documentation strategy could best be applied at the institutional level.[11] In fact, if the documentation strategy concept is to be employed, it will most successfully be employed among a group of institutions that have already embraced the concept internally.

To accentuate the distinction from the documentation strategists' call for interinstitutional planning and cooperation, the internal process advocated in this book is referred to as documentation planning. The term *documentation plan,* first used by German archivist Hans Booms to describe the proactive approach to selecting an appropriate documentary record for society,[12] was redefined almost twenty years later to apply to specific types of institution, namely, hospitals and colleges and universities.[13] In Canada the term *macro-appraisal theory* has recently arisen to refer to the underlying assumption of documentation planning: selecting documentation from the top down (i.e., beginning with an analysis of the institution's functions and the records' context) rather than from the bottom up (i.e., beginning with an examination of various record series).[14]

This book includes in the documentation planning process an additional tier of analysis, system analysis, which is an analysis of the larger system of which the institutions to be documented are a part (in this case, the U.S. health care system). The book provides background information on the U.S. health care system and the functions of the various types of institution and organization within it, thus establishing the context necessary to undertake the planning stage of the documentation planning process. Adding this analysis to a general knowledge of historical research trends, historiographic techniques, traditional appraisal criteria,[15] and a specific understanding of their institution's history, mission, culture, and resources will enable archivists to prepare effective documentation plans, thus ensuring the deliberate selection of appropriate archival materials. In addition, the overviews and typologies presented in this work will be useful to students, historians, and other researchers who need to understand and assess the "big picture" before they can focus on more specialized aspects of the U.S. health care system.

This work also describes the second element of documentation planning, the planning process, and provides as an example a portion of the documentation plan devised for Children's Hospital, Boston. The Children's Hospital documentation plan illustrates the concept of documentation planning and is, therefore, meant to be descriptive rather than prescriptive. Applying the documentation planning process and devising an actual documentation plan have not previously been attempted; therefore, the Children's Hospital documentation plan provides a necessary test case and model for other institutions, both within and outside of the health care field.

As T. R. Schellenberg noted, "analysis is the essence of archival appraisal."[16] Deciding what material to collect, the archivist's most intellectually stimulating task, has become progressively more challenging since the middle of the twentieth century because the nature of institutions and organizations has changed. In modern society, institutions are often components of multinational conglomerates or divisions of holding companies; even freestanding institutions are not truly self-contained but are linked to other institutions and organizations, both public and private, through cooperative agreements, funding arrangements, and governmental regulations. Such interconnections complicate the archivist's task by increasing the duplication of information and physically dispersing records. At the same time, more sophisticated reprographic and communications technologies have increased the quantity of records (electronic and hard copy) produced and the amount of information stored. To cope with these changes, the archival profession needs to adopt a proactive approach to documenting institutions and to pay increasing attention to the several levels of analysis underlying the archival selection process: institutional analysis, interinstitutional analysis, and system analysis.[17]

Whether or not one agrees with the need for, or efficacy of, large-scale cooperative documentation strategy initiatives, it should be clear that decisions on selecting the records of a single institution for preservation, whether by an archivist employed by that institution or by one working at a historical society or other collecting repository that has acquired a body of institutional records, should also be informed by an understanding of the place of that institution in the larger universe. Indeed, it could be argued that large-scale documentation strategies are possible only if the participating institutional archives have first come to terms with their internal issues.

Archivists can meet the challenge of documenting contemporary institutions by carefully planning what aspects of their institution they are going to document—in other words, by formulating specific plans that outline the deliberate selection of appropriate records. Documentation plans also identify functions and activities that are poorly documented, in which cases it might be desirable for the archivist to create records (e.g., oral histories) to fill in the gaps. A documentation plan is formulated in two stages, analysis and selection. The first stage consists of three tiers of analysis: (1) an institutional analysis, (2) a comparison of the institution with others of the same type, and (3) an analysis of the relationship of the institution to the larger system of which it is a part—in this case, the U.S. health care system.[18] The selection stage consists of making decisions about what to document at three levels: (1) the function, (2) the activity or project, and (3) the record series. An added benefit of documentation planning is that it increases archivists' understanding of their institutions and how they operate, which will be helpful when performing other archival activities such as processing and reference. Furthermore, the documentation planning process increases the visibility of the archives program.

Documentation planning takes a holistic or contextual approach to record selection and appraisal by adding the third and most general level of analysis to the process, thereby providing archivists with a bird's-eye view of their own institution's situation in relation to the larger systems of which they are part. When archivists are faced with the challenge of making their way through the labyrinth of appraisal, a bird's-eye view is preferable to a ground-level view. Selecting and appraising records, like mastering a labyrinth, can be accomplished more efficiently and effectively if archivists have an overview, if they carefully plan a course of action instead of making each decision as the need arises. Without this "map" or understanding of the institution in its larger context, archivists are forced to rely on luck, instinct, or precedent when making selection decisions.

Chapter 1 of this work describes the U.S. health care system in terms of its functions and the institutions and organizations that carry out those functions. Chapters 2 through 7 describe the types of institution and organization composing the health care system in terms of their functions and discusses some of the activities through which those functions are fulfilled. Because archivists are most often responsible for documenting institutions or organizations and because the U.S. health care system's structure is formed to a great extent by institutions and organizations,[19] this approach is appropriate. Furthermore, functional analysis enables archivists to work across departmental lines, which may shift, and to devise documentation plans based on what the institution does instead of how it is organized at the moment.[20] This type of analysis provides archivists with the topical, societal, and institutional contexts they need to design effective documentation plans. The analyses presented in Chapters 1 through 7 categorize and classify aspects of health care institutions, enabling archivists to select consciously which aspects to document more fully than others. Assuming that the available resources are not sufficient to document in great detail every aspect of every institution, archivists can use the analysis as a tool to assist them in making difficult decisions about which aspects to document and to what extent—in other words, to assist them in devising documentation plans.

The approach to selecting documentation presented here is suggestive rather than prescriptive. Archivists are encouraged to adapt as necessary the documentation process and plan presented in Chapter 8 to suit their specific institution. The goal is to provide the context and guidance necessary to support the development of plans for all types of institution and organization in the U.S. health care system, not to dictate what records should be preserved.

It is important for archivists to realize that the health care environment is rapidly changing. Regulations, technologies, diseases, and methods of treatment and financing are constantly evolving. Although it is not likely that the nation's health care system will be nationalized in the near future, the Clinton administration is expected to implement significant reforms. Most of these reforms will directly affect how health care delivery is financed. They may affect the configuration of health care institutions, but the functions of the U.S. health care system will remain the same.[21]

During a period of great change for the health care system, much of which is motivated by a desire to contain costs, the documentation planning process remains viable and indeed takes on special importance for health care institutions. Because the functions of the health care system will not change, they provide a base from which to gauge institutional and organizational change and on which to make archival selection decisions. As the health care system becomes more highly integrated, moreover, the emphasis of the documentation planning process on inter-institutional and system analyses also becomes more significant. With the increasing incidence of consolidations, alliances, and mergers among health care institutions and departments within these institutions, documentation planning can provide a foundation for preserving the records of emerging or reconfigured institutions and those that no longer exist.

In this new world, the traditional justifications for archival programs continue to apply. Archival programs can conserve resources by eliminating the costly storing of unnecessary records, and they can improve efficiency by providing access to important information that is needed for current institutional operations. Thus, even though the institutions and organizations described in this book will change in nature and type, the book presents a glimpse of the U.S. health care system at a particular point in time, and the concept of documentation planning and the documentation planning process remain effective tools for selecting appropriate records to document health care institutions and organizations.

NOTES

1. F. Gerald Ham, "The Archival Edge," *American Archivist* 38 (January 1975): 5–13; "Archival Strategies for the Post-Custodial Era," *American Archivist* 44 (Summer 1981): 207–16; and "Archival Choices: Managing the Historical Record in an Age of Abundance," *American Archivist* 47 (Winter 1984): 11–22.
2. The first of these was Joan Warnow et al., *A Study of Preservation of Documents at Department of Energy Laboratories* (New York: American Institute of Physics, 1982). There followed Joan K[rizack] Haas, Helen Willa Samuels, and Barbara Tripple Simmons, *Appraising the Records of Modern Science and Technology: A Guide* (Cambridge: MIT 1985; distributed by the Society of American Archivists); Bruce H. Bruemmer and Sheldon Hochheiser, *The High-Technology Company: A Historical Research and Archival Guide* (Minneapolis: Charles Babbage Institute, University of Minnesota, 1989); and *American Institute of Physics Study of Multi-Institutional Collaborations in High-Energy Physics* (New York: American Institute of Physics, 1991).
3. See, for example, Patricia Aronsson, "Appraisal of Twentieth-Century Congressional Collections," in Nancy E. Peace, ed., *Archival Choices: Managing the Historical Record in an Age of Abundance* (Lexington, Mass.: Lexington Books, 1984), 81–104; and Joan D. Krizack, "Hospital Documentation Planning: The Concept and the Context," *American Archivist* 56 (Winter 1993): 16–34. (The latter article was submitted for publication in its final form in December 1989.) Aronsson's work was recently expanded in *The Documentation of Congress: Report of the Congressional Archivists Roundtable Task Force on Congressional Documentation* (1992).

4. See Theodore R. Schellenberg's 1956 article, "The Appraisal of Modern Public Records," reprinted in Maygene F. Daniels and Timothy Walch, eds., *A Modern Archives Reader: Basic Readings on Archival Theory and Practice* (Washington, D.C.: National Archives and Records Service, 1984).
5. Helen Willa Samuels, "Who Controls the Past?" *American Archivist* 49 (Spring 1986): 109–24.
6. Ibid., 115.
7. Howard Zinn, "Secretary, Archives and the Public Interest," *Midwestern Archivist* 2 (1977): 14–26; Hans Booms, "Society and the Formation of a Documentary Heritage; Issues in the Appraisal of Archival Sources," *Archivaria* 24 (Summer 1984): 69–107 (original German version published in 1972); Ham, "The Archival Edge"; and Patrick M. Quinn, "The Archivist as Activist," *Georgia Archive* 5 (Winter 1977): 25–35.
8. Philip N. Alexander and Helen W. Samuels, "The Roots of 128: A Hypothetical Documentation Strategy," *American Archivist* 50 (Fall 1987): 518–31.
9. Richard J. Cox, "A Documentation Strategy Case Study: Western New York," *American Archivist* 52 (Spring 1989): 192–200.
10. Judith E. Endleman, "Looking Backward to Plan for the Future: Collection Analysis for Manuscript Repositories," *American Archivist* 50 (Summer 1987): 340–53; and Maureen A. Jung, "Documenting Nineteenth-Century Quartz Mining in Northern California," *American Archivist* 53 (Summer 1990): 406–18.
11. Krizack, "Hospital Documentation Planning."
12. Booms, "Society and Documentary Heritage," 105.
13. Krizack, "Hospital Documentation Planning," and Helen Willa Samuels *Varsity Letters: Documenting Modern Colleges and Universities* (Metuchen, N.J.: Society of American Archivists and Scarecrow Press, 1992).
14. For example, Richard Brown, "Records Acquisition Strategy and Its Theoretical Foundation: The Case for a Concept of Archival Hermeneutics," *Archivaria* 33 (Winter 1991–1992); 34–56; and Terry Cook, "Mind over Matter: Toward a New Theory of Archival Appraisal," in Barbara L. Craig, ed., *The Archival Imagination: Essays in Honour of Hugh A. Taylor* (Ottawa: Association of Canadian Archivists, 1992), 38–70.
15. For traditional appraisal criteria, see Schellenberg, "Modern Records," and F. Gerald Ham, *Archives and Manuscripts: Appraisal and Accessioning* (Chicago: Society of American Archivists, 1992). Also, Frank Boles and Julia Marks Young identified and categorized appraisal criteria in *Archival Appraisal* (New York: Neal-Schuman, 1991).
16. Schellenberg, "Modern Public Records," 68.
17. It should be noted that Schellenberg was writing about governmental archives and referring to the need for analysis at the agency and record series levels.
18. This is not a new idea; it is an extension of the strategy for appraising governmental records advocated by Theodore R. Schellenberg in *Modern Archives: Principles and Techniques* (Chicago: University of Chicago Press, 1956), 52.

19. Milton I. Roemer, *Ambulatory Health Services in America: Past, Present, and Future* (Rockville, Md.: Aspen Publishers, 1981), 30.
20. For a more detailed explanation of functional analysis and its value, see Helen Willa Samuels, "Rationale for the Functional Approach," in *Varsity Letters: Documenting Modern Colleges and Universities* (Metuchen, N.J.: Scarecrow Press, 1992), 1–18.
21. For more specific information on impending health care reforms, see Chapter 2.

DOCUMENTATION PLANNING FOR THE U.S. HEALTH CARE SYSTEM

CHAPTER 1

Overview of the U.S. Health Care System

JOAN D. KRIZACK

The U.S. health care system is complex and constantly changing. Since World War II, it has grown to become one of the two largest American industries. In 1992 the nation spent $838.5 billion, or 14 percent of the gross national product, on health care—a higher proportion than that spent by any other country. Compared to other nations' systems, health care in the United States is decentralized and competitive, characterized by a mix of public and private health care institutions and organizations.[1] In fact, the United States is one of only two developed countries (the other is the Republic of South Africa) that does not have a health care system run by its government.

If a health care system is defined as "a group of curative and preventative service components—organized, coordinated, and controlled to achieve certain goals,"[2] then the U.S. health care system may be more accurately described as a nonsystem, largely because of the predominance of free enterprise and the absence of nationalized health care.[3] It is, nevertheless, stable and resilient, both because it is decentralized and diverse and because the medical profession itself exercises tremendous power through organizations such as the American Medical Association. The government's role is also powerful and is primarily exercised through governmental regulation, especially regarding third-party payment mechanisms and health care standards.

Broadly viewed, the health care system has six major functions:

- patient care (diagnosis and treatment)
- health promotion (activities aimed at encouraging good health, such as fitness programs and informational campaigns)

- biomedical research
- education (of health care professionals)
- regulation and formulation of policy (*regulation* establishes standards for institutions and practitioners; *formulation of policy* involves coordinating health care services within a specified region or jurisdiction on a suprainstitutional level)
- provision of goods and services (such as pharmaceuticals, wheelchairs, diagnostic and therapeutic equipment, and malpractice and health insurance)

These functions are carried out by diverse institutions and organizations that interact and overlap with one another, each institution encompassing one or more functions in its mission (sometimes along with other functions that are not related to health care). The institutions may be classified as:

- health care delivery facilities (e.g., hospitals, nursing homes, hospices),
- health agencies and foundations (e.g., U.S. Department of Health and Human Services, Robert Wood Johnson Foundation),
- biomedical research facilities (e.g., Boston Biomedical Research Institute; Acupuncture Institute, Monterey, California),
- educational institutions for the health professions (e.g., Massachusetts College of Pharmacy and Allied Health Sciences, Forsyth Dental Center School for Dental Hygienists, Bowman Gray School of Medicine),
- professional and voluntary associations (e.g., American Nurses Association, American College of Healthcare Executives, American Cancer Society), and
- health industries (e.g., Merck, Codman and Shurtleff, Johnson & Johnson, Blue Cross/Blue Shield).[4]

These institutions are funded by governments, voluntary contributions, investors, philanthropic foundations (notably the W. K. Kellogg, Robert Wood Johnson, and Rockefeller foundations), or by a combination of these methods.[5]

The matrix depicted in Table 1–1 is a visual representation of the conjunction of the health care system's functions and organizations. Although the matrix is artificial and contrived, it provides archivists with an overview of an extremely complex system in terms that are meaningful to their work.

Brief descriptions of the six categories of health care institutions and organizations follow. In-depth studies of each category are provided in Chapters 2 through 7.

TABLE 1–1 The U.S. health care system: an archival perspective

	Functions of the U.S. Health Care System					
Institutions and Organizations	**Health Care Delivery**		Biomedical Research	Education	Regulation/ Policy Formulation	Provision of Goods/ Services
	Patient Care	Health Promotion				
Delivery facilities	1	2	2	2		
Agencies/foundations	2	1	2	2	1	
Research facilities	2		1	2		
Educational institutions	2	2	1	1		
Professional/voluntary associations	2	1	2	1	1	
Health industries		2	1			1

1 = primary function, 2 = secondary function.

HEALTH CARE DELIVERY FACILITIES

Health care delivery facilities are numerous and varied, but the most important are hospitals, which account for 44 percent of all health care dollars spent.[6] Although their major function is to provide patient care, some facilities, including hospitals, are also involved in three of the other five functions of the health care system: health promotion, biomedical research, and education.

Two general categories of health care facility exist: ambulatory care facilities (which offer a range of services from routine treatment and counseling to relatively complex services for conditions that do not warrant hospitalization) and in-patient facilities. Some facilities, notably hospitals, provide both ambulatory and in-patient services, and some hospitals run satellite outpatient clinics. Physicians' offices, clinics, health maintenance organizations (which, like Kaiser Permanente, may also own hospitals),[7] hospital emergency rooms and outpatient departments, and freestanding, for-profit "emergicenters" or "surgicenters" are settings for ambulatory care.

Physicians' offices may house a single physician or a group of physicians in private practice; the trend today is toward group practice.[8] Physicians may also see private patients in an office located in or near a hospital. Public health clinics are open to all in need of health services but predominantly serve individuals with lower incomes or without health insurance.[9] Clinics are numerous and diverse, consisting of government sponsored clinics (public health agency clinics, neighborhood health centers), special voluntary clinics (family planning or cancer detection clinics), for-profit outpatient clinics (Healthstop, located in the Boston area and elsewhere), and clinics within institutions such as elementary and secondary schools, colleges and universities, prisons, industries, and businesses. Limited outpatient health services may also be provided in the patient's home by private nurses and other health care professionals, for-profit health care businesses, voluntary agencies (the Visiting Nurses Association), hospitals, and hospices.

In-patient care is provided in nursing homes, hospices, freestanding birthing centers, substance abuse facilities, and hospitals. With the exception of nursing homes, these facilities may also provide outpatient care.

HEALTH AGENCIES AND FOUNDATIONS

Health agencies, one of the most complex and diverse components of the U.S. health care system, may be public or voluntary agencies. Public health care agencies exist at all levels of government—federal, state, and local. At the federal level, the government is involved in all six of the functions defined above. The federal government plays a direct role in the delivery of health care (for example, through Veterans Administration hospitals), but it also has an indirect role, providing funding and delegating authority to public and private institutions or organizations to carry out primary health care activities.[10] Recently, the federal government has become less involved in providing patient care and more involved in funding it.[11] Although the federal government is involved in biomedical research, educating health care professionals, and promoting health, its primary roles are in funding health care services and in regulation and policy formulation, especially through the Food and Drug Administration. The Department of Health and Human Services is responsible for most federal activity related to health care. It is subdivided into four major units: the Health Care Financing Administration, which oversees the Medicare and Medicaid programs, setting standards for care; the Social Security Administration; the Administration for Children and Families; and the Public Health Service, which engages in a broad range of general and specialized health care activities.

The Public Health Service, in turn, comprises eight agencies: the Substance Abuse and Mental Health Services Administration; the Centers for Disease Control; the Food and Drug Administration; the Health Resources and Services Administration, which is the primary focus for the federal government's patient care programs and administers the Gillis W. Long Hansen's Disease Center in Louisiana; the Agency for Toxic Substances and Disease Registry; the National Institutes of Health, which includes fourteen research institutes, one hospital, and several centers and divisions; the Indian Health Service, which provides health care services to native Americans and Alaskan natives; and the Agency for Health Care Policy and Research.[12]

This sketch outlines only part of the federal government's role in the health care system. Other governmental agencies outside the Department of Health and Human Services have health care responsibilities as part of their missions. All branches of the U.S. military, for example, run hospitals for their employees, the Department of Transportation operates Coast Guard hospitals (which are staffed by Public Health Service staff), and the Department of Veterans Affairs is responsible for approximately 170 hospitals, the country's largest network of public hospitals.[13] The Defense Department also administers the Uniformed Services University of the Health Sciences and conducts extensive programs of biomedical research.

Although the federal government plays a significant role in the health care system, the ultimate responsibility for the health and welfare of the general public and the legal authority in health care matters rest with the states.[14] To this end, each state has an agency responsible for health care, but it is important to understand that there is significant variation in their roles. The missions of state health care agencies include five of the six functions of the health care system. These agencies are involved in formulating state-wide policy, administering programs that receive federal funds, such as Medicaid. They are also involved in regulation through licensing health professionals and facilities, establishing rate-setting commissions for hospitals, and providing safety codes for housing, institutions, and industry. The states educate and train health professionals through formal programs in state colleges and universities. They also engage in biomedical research, which outside of the college and universities setting is usually epidemiological in nature. States promote health and work to prevent illness by monitoring, for example, the quality of food and water supplies and by communicable disease control. States also provide patient care through institutions for people with mental or emotional difficulties, people with developmental disabilities, and chronically ill people, among others. In some states it is difficult to distinguish state from local patient care.

The primary functions of local health agencies are the coordination and regulation of health care services at the local level and the delivery of health care; however, the range of activities within these functions varies greatly from state to state. Local health departments record and analyze health data, work to prevent illness by educating the public in health matters, provide environmental health services, and administer health services through the operation of health care facilities. Usually these services are limited to activities such as immunization, well-baby examinations, and screening for chronic diseases, but sometimes they cover the full range of health care services. Local health departments may also provide school health services.[15]

Foundations, which may be defined as organizations that exist to distribute private funds to nonprofit institutions and organizations, also play a key role in the health care system.[16] Local foundations may support neighborhood hospitals, while national foundations support biomedical research (e.g., the W. K. Kellogg Foundation), medical education (the Rockefeller Foundation), and policy formulation (the Commonwealth Fund). They exert significant influence on health care policy through policy studies and through their funding decisions.

BIOMEDICAL RESEARCH FACILITIES

Biomedical research takes place in laboratories, departments, and institutions involved in pursuing knowledge related to health care. Research facilities may be freestanding (e.g., the Worcester Foundation for Experimental Biology) or part of another institution such as a hospital (the Eaton Peabody Laboratory of Auditory Physiology at the Massachusetts Eye and Ear Infirmary), academic health center, industry, and the federal government. Biomedical research laboratories in hospitals may be sponsored by outside organizations such as medical schools, private foundations, or voluntary health agencies. Biomedical research takes place both in institutions whose sole function is investigative work and, more often, in institutions in which research is only one of several functions (for example, teaching hospitals).

EDUCATIONAL INSTITUTIONS FOR THE HEALTH PROFESSIONS

There are thirty-five major categories of health care profession in the U.S. health care system.[17] Membership in each of these professions requires specific training, ranging from in-house training for nurses' aides and orderlies to postdoctoral training for medical specialists and subspecialists. Institutions involved in educating health professionals may have this as their primary function (e.g., the Massachusetts College of Pharmacy and Allied Health Sciences, and the Forsyth Dental Center School for Dental Hygienists) or it may be one of a number of functions, as is the case for teaching hospitals. Educational programs for many health care professionals, including physicians, nurses, medical records personnel, dental hygienists, and laboratory technicians, are offered by technical high schools, colleges or universities, and for-profit educational organizations.

Education for certain health professionals occurs wholly or in part in hospitals. In the past, most nurses were trained in hospital-based programs, but recently many of these programs have been phased out. Now nurses also receive degrees from academic institutions. Although universities are the major site for physician education, hospitals are the setting for physicians' extensive clinical training. Teaching hospitals[18] are most often owned by universities, medical schools, or an umbrella organization. In some cases the teaching hospital and medical school have a formal affiliation that does not include ownership. Recently, some academic institutions have formed holding companies that control their hospitals.

Hospitals also provide continuing education for health professionals. In the case of nurses and physicians, for example, continuing education programs are regularly offered to enable these professionals to maintain licensure or be relicensed. Continuing education programs may also be sponsored by professional associations, universities, or corporations outside the hospital setting.

PROFESSIONAL AND VOLUNTARY ASSOCIATIONS

All health care professions have professional associations. Their major function is education, and they may also engage in accreditation or certification activities. Many of these societies are also involved in formulating policy and regulating health care services, mainly through legislative lobbying efforts. Some associations are national in scope; regional or local associations may be independent or branches of national groups. Professional associations are funded for the most part by membership dues. Some of the larger national associations maintain administrative headquarters, which are often centrally located in the Midwest. (The American Medical Association and the American College of Healthcare Executives, among others, are headquartered in Chicago.) The purpose of these associations is to advance the specific profession in the health care field; to elevate professional standards through accreditation or certifica-

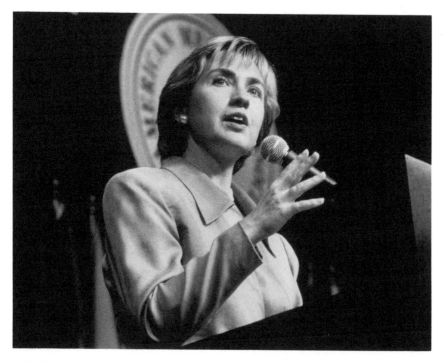

FIGURE 1–1 Hillary Rodham Clinton, chair of the president's Task Force on National Health Reform, addressing the American Medical Association's House of Delegates, 1993. *Source:* American Medical Association

tion activities; to provide pertinent information, usually through meetings, newsletters, and journals; and to protect the profession's interests by legislative lobbying.[19]

Voluntary associations also play an important role in the U.S. health care system. These associations support biomedical research and sometimes provide health care services to individuals; in most instances, however, their most important function is to educate the public.[20] Their funding comes from private and corporate contributions, subscription fees, and fund-raising events. These associations may be concerned with a specific disease or organ (for example, the American Cancer Society and the American Heart Association), the health of special groups (Planned Parenthood Federation of America, the National Easter Seal Society for Crippled Adults and Children), certain types of health service (the Visiting Nurses Association, which provides home health care), or health policy (the National Health Council and the National Safety Council).[21] Some voluntary associations are not primarily related to health but are involved in the health care system. Fraternal organizations, for example, may fund medical research (the Lions Club funds eye research) or run nonprofit hospitals (the Shriners sponsor children's specialty hospitals).

HEALTH INDUSTRIES

Companies providing goods and services related to health care delivery support the basic patient care function of the U.S. health care system. In addition, some companies, particularly pharmaceutical companies, are involved in biomedical research. Health industries include pharmaceutical companies; hospital supply companies, which produce disposable products such as syringes, surgical drapes, and sterile gloves; companies that manufacture appliances, including wheelchairs and prosthetic devices; pharmacies; and companies that manufacture diagnostic instruments (for example, x-ray machines and other imaging systems) or therapeutic equipment (such as incubators and lasers). Some companies provide services, for example, clinical laboratory tests, laundry service, management expertise, and health insurance.

THE CHANGING NATURE OF THE U.S. HEALTH CARE SYSTEM

As noted in the Introduction, some reforms in the U.S. health care system are expected during the Clinton administration. Although the reforms will not result in a national health program and the system will remain distinctly American, significant changes will be legislated. These changes which are focused on insurance reform will affect payment mechanisms, and they may affect the nature of health care institutions and organizations composing the U.S. health care system, but they will not affect the functions of the broader system.

Reform of the nation's health care system is being undertaken in a effort to control costs and extend basic health care coverage to the 37 million Americans who are without health insurance. Hospitals, health maintenance organizations, and other health care delivery facilities will continue to be subject to financial pressures aimed at controlling costs. To remain competitive in the marketplace, they are merging, combining services, or forming alliances. The merger of Columbia Healthcare Corporation and Galen Health Care Inc. in late 1993, for example, and the subsequent merger with HCA-Hospital Corporation of America created the largest chain of for-profit hospitals in the country. The new entity, Columbia Healthcare Corporation, owns one-hundred ninety hospitals in twenty-six states and two foreign countries.[22] Not-for-profit hospitals are also redefining themselves. In the Boston area, for example, Boston University Medical Center, the New England Deaconess Hospital, and Massachusetts General Hospital, among others, are shaping alliances with hospitals in southeastern Massachusetts to increase their patient bases; community hospitals north of the city have merged to create a more efficient, competitive system; and five Harvard Medical School–affiliated teaching hospitals have formed the Harvard Medical Planning Group, under the leadership of the medical school's dean, to discuss a cooperative strategy for eliminating duplicated medical services.[23]

Other health care institutions will be affected by health care reform. Because the government will play an even stronger regulatory role, governmental agencies will evolve, though national and state responsibilities remain to be sorted out. At this point, too, it is not clear how research facilities and educational institutions will be affected. Academic health centers—where health care delivery, research, and education are joined—cannot provide health care services as inexpensively as other health care delivery facilities, and they are concerned about maintaining a competitive edge while engaging in education and research.[24] It is almost certain that in the new atmosphere that stresses efficiency and cost control, emphasis will be placed on educating primary care physicians and researching topics related to primary care. The health industries will undoubtedly be affected by price constraints if not controls, and alliances are already forming between health industries and hospitals. For example, Baxter International Inc., the world's largest hospital supply company, and American Healthcare Systems, one of the largest hospital groups in the United States, have reached an agreement covering medical and surgical supplies that American will purchase from Baxter.[25] The health insurance industry may be transformed into a few giant companies that negotiate services for large groups of clients or into companies that manage networks of health care providers. Professional and voluntary associations are the organizations least likely to be directly affected by health care reform, but the altered system will mean significant changes for at least some of them.

NOTES

1. J. Rogers Hollingsworth, *A Political Economy of Medicine: Great Britain and the United States* (Baltimore: Johns Hopkins University Press, 1986), 3, 163.
2. James M. Rosser and Howard E. Mossberg, *An Analysis of Health Care Delivery* (New York: John Wiley & Sons, 1977), 1.
3. Milton I. Roemer, *An Introduction to the U.S. Health Care System* (New York: Springer Publishing Company, 1986), 2.
4. Adapted from Rosser and Mossberg, *Health Care Delivery*, 24–63, and Roemer, *U.S. Health Care System*, 5–12.
5. This book deals with the U.S. health care system in institutional terms. Therefore, folk medicine provided by friends or relatives in the home and health promotion activities, such as exercise classes that are conducted outside the institutional structures outlined here, are not covered by this work. Veterinary education and research, however, are included because they are integrated within the U.S. health care institutions as defined above.
6. ''Is the Business of Medicine Business?'' *New York Times Book Review*, 5 April 1992, 11.
7. A health maintenance organization (HMO) is a comprehensive system of therapeutic and preventative health services that are provided to an enrolled population for a fixed per-person sum.
8. Russel C. Coile, Jr., *The New Medicine: Reshaping Medical Practice and Health Care Management* (Rockville, Md.: Aspen Publishers, 1990), 240.
9. Stephen J. Williams and Paul R. Torrens, *Introduction to Health Services* (New York: John Wiley & Sons, 1984), 164.
10. Roemer, *U.S. Health Care System*, 6.
11. Anthony R. Kovner, and contributors, *Health Care Delivery in the United States*, 4th ed. (New York: Springer Publishing Company, 1990), 306.
12. United States Government Manual, 1989–90 (Washington, D.C.: U.S. Government Printing Office, 1990).
13. Williams and Torrens, *Introduction to Health Services*, 172.
14. Joellen Watson Hawkins and Loretta Pierfedeici Higgins, *Nursing and the American Health Care Delivery System* (New York: Tiresias Press, 1982), 34.
15. Rosser and Mossberg, *Health Care Delivery*, 28, and Kovner, *Health Care Delivery*, 123.

16. *The Foundation Directory* (New York: Foundation Center, 1989), Introduction.
17. Hawkins and Higgins, *Nursing,* 111.
18. See page 33 for the definition of a teaching hospital.
19. Rosser and Mossberg, *Health Care Delivery,* 33–34.
20. Hawkins and Higgins, *Nursing,* 45.
21. Adapted from Roemer, *U.S. Health Care System,* 9, and Rosser and Mossberg, *Health Care Delivery,* 29, 32–33.
22. "The Hospital World's Hard-Driving Money Man," *New York Times,* 5 October, 1993, D1.
23. The five are Beth Israel, Brigham and Women's, Children's, Massachusetts General, and New England Deaconess hospitals.
24. For more information on academic health centers, see Chapter 5.
25. "A $4 Billion Supply Deal for Hospitals" *New York Times,* 26 Oct 1993.

ANNOTATED SELECTED BIBLIOGRAPHY

For an excellent history of medicine in the United States,see Paul Starr, *The Social Transformation of American Medicine: The Rise of a Sovereign Profession and the Making of a Vast Industry* (New York: Basic Books, 1982). This volume, which won the 1984 Pulitzer Prize for general nonfiction, traces the origins of medical practice through the growth of corporate medicine, from 1760 to 1980.

A highly recommended source that describes the basic elements of the U.S. health care system and their interaction is Anthony R. Kovner, and contributors *Health Care Delivery in the United States,* 4th ed. (New York: Springer Publishing Company, 1990).

Other good sources that describe the U.S. health care system include Steven Jonas, *An Introduction to the U.S. Health Care System* (New York: Springer Publishing Company, 1992) and David Barton Smith and Arnold D. Kaluzny, *The White Labyrinth: A Guide to the Health Care System* (Ann Arbor, Mich.: Health Administration Press, 1986). "Historical Evolution and Overview of Health Services in the United States," chapter 1 in Stephen J. Williams and Paul R. Torrens, *Introduction to Health Services* (New York: Wiley, 1984), describes the types of health care program within the system as a whole.

Although somewhat dated, a valuable source comparing the U.S. health care system with the systems of other countries is Marshall W. Raffel, ed., *Comparative Health Systems: Discriptive Analysis of Fourteen National Health Systems* (University Park: Pennsylvania State University Press, 1984). Another source that compares health care systems is J. Rogers Hollingsworth, *A Political Economy of Medicine: Great Britain and the United States* (Baltimore: Johns Hopkins University Press, 1986). Chapter 2, "The Medical Delivery System of the U. S., 1890–1970," provides a good historical overview with comparisons made to England and Wales.

CHAPTER 2

Facilities That Deliver Health Care

JOAN D. KRIZACK

The delivery of health care, which may be defined as the provision of diagnostic and therapeutic services to individuals and the promotion of good health, is the primary function of the U.S. health care system. Like the system itself, it involves a complex mix of institutions, organizations, and individuals and a variety of public and private sponsors.

Institutions that deliver health care may be classified according to whether they offer in-patient care, ambulatory (outpatient) care, or both. (See Tables 2–1 and 2–2 for a typology of health care delivery settings.) In-patient care is care given to a patient confined to an institution overnight or longer. Most in-patient care is provided in a hospital; however, free-standing birthing centers, hospices, nursing homes, prison and school infirmaries, and substance abuse facilities may also offer in-patient care. Ambulatory care is generally understood to refer to health care provided to individuals not confined to a hospital.[1] Because governmental regulations limit reimbursement for Medicare and Medicaid patients and because other third-party payers are implementing cost-containing rules, ambulatory care services are expanding to include procedures that formerly were performed only on an in-patient basis. Some institutions, including most hospitals, provide ambulatory services in addition to in-patient care. (See Table 2–2 for a typology of ambulatory care clinics.)

Hospitals, which have been described as "the center of both medical practice and the experience of illness,"[2] are the institutional focus of the U.S. health care system. For this reason, and because the functions and activities of a hospital parallel those that occur in other in-patient and

TABLE 2–1 Typology of health care delivery settings

In-Patient Care Settings
Birthing centers
Hospices
Hospitals
Nursing homes
Secondary school, college, and university infirmaries
Substance abuse programs

Ambulatory Care Settings
Private physician offices
   Solo practice
   Group practice
      General/family practice group
      Single specialty
      Multispecialty
Institutional settings
   Business/industry
   Health maintenance organizations
   Holistic health centers
   Hospitals
   Prisons
   Private homes
   Schools
Freestanding clinics (see Table 2–2)

ambulatory settings, this chapter will concentrate on hospitals. A brief discussion of other in-patient and ambulatory care settings, focusing on their distinctive characteristics, follows the discussion of hospitals.

HOSPITALS

Of all the institutions that engage in the delivery of health care, hospitals are the most central to the U.S. health care system. With the increasing use of expensive medical technology in both diagnosis and treatment, the hospital has become the central health care institution in the United States. In 1990 the number of hospitals in the United States was 6,649[3] (as compared to 3,535 institutions of higher education),[4] and $256 billion was spent on hospital services (almost 39 percent of the $666.2 billion spent on health care).[5]

TABLE 2–2   Typology of ambulatory clinics

According to Clientele Served
Clinics for Alaskan natives
Clinics for native Americans
Clinics for military personnel and their dependents
Clinics for poor people
Geriatric clinics
Migrant worker health clinics
Maternal and infant clinics
Neighborhood/community clinics ("free" clinics)
Rural clinics
Teen clinics
Women's clinics

According to Condition(s) Diagnosed/Treated
AIDS and HIV clinics
Ambulatory surgery centers
Arthritis clinics
Birthing centers
Cancer detection centers
Dental clinics
Diabetes clinics
Diagnostic imaging centers
Dialysis centers
Emergency (urgent) care clinics (emergicenters)
Family planning clinics
Heart disease clinics
Immunization clinics
Mental health clinics
Obstetrics and gynecology clinics
Pain relief clinics
Primary care clinics
Rehabilitation centers (cardiac, physical)
Sexually transmitted or venereal disease clinics
Sports injury clinics
Substance abuse clinics
Surgicenters
Tuberculosis screening clinics
Vision disorder clinics

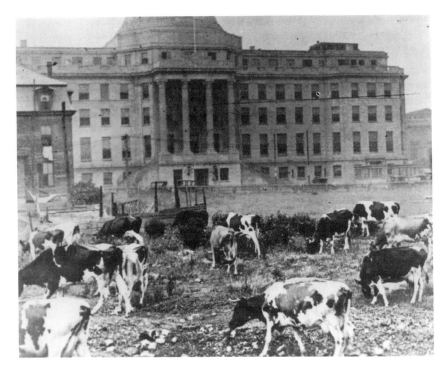

FIGURE 2-1　The Hunnewell Building of Children's Hospital, Boston, circa 1919. Milk from the cows in the foreground was pasteurized in the hospital's Milk Laboratory and given to patients to prevent them from contracting bovine tuberculosis. *Source:* Children's Hospital Archives

Hospitals were not always the focus of medical practice, education, and research that they are today. In the eighteenth and nineteenth centuries, poor people who were sick went to hospitals, while the middle and upper classes received medical care at home. With the introduction of antisepsis, however, hospitals became safer, and since the early twentieth century they have become indispensable to providing medical care, educating health care professionals, and conducting biomedical research.[6]

Hospitals perform four of the six functions of the U.S. health care system defined in Chapter 1. In addition to the patient care, education, and biomedical research functions, many hospitals have health promotion programs, although it should be noted that historically, the U.S. health care system has emphasized treatment over prevention. Regulation is not a function of hospitals, which are themselves regulated by federal, state, and local governmental agencies. Neither are they involved in health care policy formulation. Hospitals do, however, influence health care policy and regulation mainly through the lobbying activities of state hospital associations and the American Hospital Association.

TYPES OF HOSPITAL

A hospital may be broadly defined as a health care treatment facility with six or more in-patient beds.[7] Hospitals in the Unites States compose a heterogeneous, decentralized, and fragmented grouping of institutions about which it is extremely difficult to generalize. Nevertheless, it is important to attempt to categorize them and describe their similarities and differences, thus providing a broad context within which archivists can construct documentation plans. As with most efforts at classification, some hospitals cannot neatly be placed into one category (mobile hospitals), and some fit equally well into more than one category (women's and children's hospitals).

For the purpose of this study, hospitals are categorized in terms of five characteristics: (1) ownership or control, (2) degree of independence, (3) the type of patient treated or services provided, (4) whether or not the hospital is involved in educating or training health care professionals, and (5) whether or not the hospital is involved in biomedical research. (See Tables 2–3 and 2–4.) The first three characteristics are the most important from an archival standpoint because they have the greatest impact on the types of record created and where the records are located. If a hospital engages in educational activities and/or biomedical research, the types of record created will obviously reflect these activities; conversely, if a hospital does not engage in education and research, no records reflecting these activities will exist. Because the patterns of hospital ownership and control are relatively diverse and complex (see Table 2–4), as are the various configurations in which a hospital is part of a larger organization, they are described in detail below.

Ownership or Control: Government The federal government, most state governments, and many local governments own and operate hospitals. In 1991 the federal government ran 5 percent of the nation's hospitals; state and local governments operated 26 percent.

In the *federal government* the organization most directly concerned with health care is the Department of Health and Human Services (DHHS). The division of the DHHS most directly concerned with the delivery of health care is the Public Health Service, which in turn comprises eight agencies. Within the Public Health Service, for example, the Substance Abuse and Mental Health Services Administration jointly administers, with the District of Columbia, St. Elizabeths Hospital, in Washington,

TABLE 2–3 Typology of hospitals

Ownership/Control (see Table 2–4)

Degree of Independence
Freestanding
Larger organization
 Health care company
 Health maintenance organization
 Holding company
 Multihospital system or chain
 Part of a university, industry, business

Patients Treated or Services Provided
Type of patient treated
 Black hospitals
 Geriatric hospitals and nursing homes
 Hospitals for employees of specific businesses/industries
 Hospitals serving native Americans/Alaskan natives
 Military hospitals
 Pediatric hospitals
 Prison hospitals
 School/university infirmaries
 Veterans hospitals
 Women's hospitals (women's and children's hospitals are sometimes
  combined)
Type of service provided
 Alcohol/drug abuse hospitals
 Burn hospitals
 Cancer hospitals
 Chronic disease hospitals/hospices
 Communicable diseases hospitals
 Convalescent hospitals
 Diabetes hospitals
 Epilepsy hospitals
 Eye, ear, nose, and throat hospitals
 Eye hospitals
 General medical and surgical hospitals
 Homeopathic hospitals
 Hospitals for mentally retarded people
 Immunology and respiratory (including tuberculosis) hospitals
 Leprosaria
 Maternity hospitals
 Orthopedic hospitals
 Osteopathic hospitals
 Physical rehabilitation hospitals
 Psychiatric hospitals

Hospital Engages in Education

Hospital Engages in Research

TABLE 2–4 Hospital ownership or control

Governmental Ownership
Federal
  Department of Defense
    Air Force
    Army
    Navy
  Department of Health and Human Services, Public Health Service
    Health Resources and Services Administration
    Indian Health Service
    National Institutes of Health, Clinical Center
  Department of Justice, Bureau of Prisons
  Department of Transportation, U.S. Coast Guard
  Department of Veterans Affairs
State
  State health agencies (long-term facilities for chronically ill, people with
    developmental disabilities, and people with mental or emotional
    difficulties)
  State prison/reformatory hospitals
  State university medical school hospitals
Local
  City/county joint hospitals
  City hospitals
  County hospitals
  District hospitals

Private Ownership
Voluntary (nonprofit)
  Business/industry
  Church or religious order
  Community group
  Fraternal organization
  Health care cooperative/collective
  Health maintenance organization
  Private university
Proprietary (for profit)
  Corporation
  Individual owner
  Partnership

D.C., which is a psychiatric hospital for residents of the District of Columbia and the Virgin Islands; the Health Resources and Services Administration provides health care services to Hansen's disease (leprosy) patients and others at the Gillis W. Long Hansen's Disease Center, in Carville, Louisiana; the Indian Health Service runs 50 hospitals and more than 300 clinics for native Americans and Alaskan natives[8]; and the National Institutes of Health's Warren Grant Magnuson Clinical Center consists of a 540-bed hospital and laboratory complex.[9]

Other departments of the federal government are also involved in the delivery of health care. The Department of Defense, for example, controls army, navy, and air force hospitals, both in this country and abroad, providing health care services to military personnel and their dependents. Through the Department of Veterans Affairs, the federal government also operates approximately 170 veterans hospitals, the majority of which are general hospitals but some of which are psychiatric hospitals. The Department of Justice, Bureau of Prisons, Health Services Division, provides health care services for prisoners in federal institutions and runs the Medical Center for Federal Prisoners, a large referral hospital. The Department of Transportation runs U.S. Coast Guard hospitals in Kodiak, Alaska, and New London, Connecticut.

State governments operate long-term facilities providing care for people with mental or emotional difficulties and people with developmental disabilities; in 1991 250 state mental hospitals were in operation, though the patient population was reduced only a fraction of what it had been a generation earlier. State prison, state reformatory, and state university medical school hospitals (for example, the University Hospital at the University of Michigan Medical School) are controlled to some extent by state governments. Historically, states also ran hospitals for tuberculosis patients (Glenridge Hospital, Glenville, New York, for example, which closed in 1978).

Local governments, embodied in districts, counties, and cities, may also run hospitals. In 1991 local governments controlled 1,393 hospitals (1,352 general, 15 psychiatric, and 26 other), or 21 percent of all U.S. hospitals. District hospitals, found in a few states, including California, are governed by boards of directors who are elected by district residents; county hospitals are generally run by county boards of supervisors (for example, Cook County Hospital, Chicago); and city hospitals are owned by municipal governments and managed by appointed boards of citizens (Boston City Hospital). Sometimes city and county governments jointly control a hospital.

Most public hospitals were founded to provide health care to indigent people who were not served by voluntary hospitals. Today, public hospitals include teaching hospitals, a small number of large general hospitals treating primarily indigent people, some hospitals in urban areas in which the patient profile is similar to that in voluntary hospitals, and many small, rural hospitals.[10]

Ownership or Control: Private The sizable number of voluntary hospitals was born of the country's ethnic and religious diversity.[11] Historically, *voluntary* or *nonprofit* hospitals were established by community leaders or by religious or ethnic groups to serve the "deserving poor" and individuals who became ill while away from home. Voluntary hospitals provided free care and were paternalistic toward their patients. As a rule, however, they did not treat indigent, contagious, morally lacking, mentally ill, or chronically ill patients; this task was left to public hospitals.[12]

Voluntary hospitals, which accounted for 51 percent of U.S. hospitals in 1991, are owned and/or operated by seven types of organization: (1) churches or religious groups (including Baptist, Lutheran, and Roman Catholic churches, the Salvation Army, the Sisters of Mercy, and the Alexian Brothers); (2) private universities (e.g., Boston University's University Hospital); (3) fraternal organizations (the Shriners); (4) industry (railroad and lumber companies); (5) community groups composed of citizens who organize to provide health care for their community and make annual contributions (Beth Israel Hospital, Boston)[13]; (6) health maintenance organizations (Kaiser Foundation Health Plan, Inc.); and (7) cooperatives, which are owned by those who use their services (Group Health Cooperative of Puget Sound).[14]

Proprietary or *for-profit* hospitals are usually set up as partnerships or corporations. They emerged where community groups could not raise the funds necessary to establish voluntary hospitals. In the late nineteenth century and well into the twentieth century physicians often owned hospitals because it was convenient to have a hospital close to their offices. Furthermore, by starting their own hospital, physicians who did not have admitting privileges in existing hospitals could treat patients needing hospitalization instead of referring them to a colleague. Such physician-owned hospitals, once common, are now rare.

During the Depression, many proprietary hospitals were closed or merged with voluntary or public hospitals. After the passage of Medicare and Medicaid legislation in 1965, however, the number of proprietary hospitals rose again, because they were now reimbursed for interest on their debt, plant depreciation, and capital equipment.[15] After for-profit hospitals were reimbursed by the government for Medicare and Medicaid patients, they became more like voluntary hospitals. At the same time, voluntary hospitals became more like for-profit hospitals because the government reimbursed them for some of their charity work.

Before 1965, the American public held a strong prejudice against the for-profit hospital sector because the practice of medicine was viewed as charity or a service to humanity. This prejudice lessened to some extent once voluntary and proprietary hospitals became more like each other.[16] Proprietary hospitals, however, continue to lag behind the hospital industry as a whole in conducting research and providing outpatient services, emergency services, health promotion services, and education for medical professionals.[17]

For the past several years, the number of proprietary hospitals has remained stable.[18] In 1991, 17.5 percent of hospitals were proprietary, representing a decrease of 0.4 percent since 1950; however, the number of beds and admissions in proprietary hospitals both increased significantly during this period.

Degree of Independence   Whether a hospital is freestanding or part of a larger organization is important to understanding where documentation is located. Obviously, if the hospital is freestanding there are fewer possibilities than if it is part of a larger organization. There are several configurations for a hospital within a larger organization. A hospital may be one of the institutions composing a *holding company.* The Massachusetts Eye and Ear Infirmary, for example, is part of the Foundation of the Massachusetts Eye and Ear Infirmary, which is an umbrella organization made up of the nonprofit infirmary and the Circle Company, a for-profit real estate company that owns a hotel and a parking garage with several storefronts. A few *health maintenance organizations* (HMOs) own one or more hospitals. An example is Kaiser Permanente, which owns more than twenty-five.[19] Hospitals are also owned by *health care corporations,* such as National Medical Enterprises, Inc., which in 1992 owned thirty-six general hospitals, thirty-two rehabilitation hospitals, seventy-five psychiatric hospitals and substance abuse facilities, eighty-five nursing homes, and thirty-five diagnostic centers in the United States, in addition to hospitals in Australia, Great Britain, Spain, and Singapore.[20]

Multihospital systems are three or more voluntary hospitals (e.g., Adventist Health System) or governmental hospitals (e.g., Veterans Administration hospitals) that collaborate through ownership, management, or lease arrangements to enhance patient care. Their for-profit counterparts are hospital chains such as Columbia Healthcare Corporation, which was founded in 1985 by Richard L. Scott and merged in 1993 with Galem Health Care and HCA-Hospital Corporation of America, creating a network of one hundred ninety hospitals in twenty-six states and two foreign countries.[21] In 1986 one third of all U.S. hospitals were divisions of multihospital systems.[22]

Finally, hospitals may be part of a *university* (there are 45 public university hospitals in the United States), *industry*, or *business*. The University Hospital in Boston, for example, is owned by Boston University; and at the turn of the century many of the larger railroad, mining, and lumbering companies built, owned, and operated hospitals for their employees.[23] With the dramatic rise in the cost of operating health care facilities and the increased availability of group health insurance, company-owned hospitals are no longer common; however, in an attempt to hold down rising health care costs, several large corporations are establishing in-house clinics and pharmacies for their employees.[24]

REGIONAL PATTERNS

Certain patterns of hospital ownership and control are more prevalent in some areas of the country than in others. Proprietary hospitals were begun in areas where the population was too poor or too scattered to support a voluntary hospital. The majority of proprietary hospitals, therefore, are located in the South, West, and Southwest[25]; California, Texas, Florida, and Tennessee claim the most.[26] Voluntary hospitals are still most prevalent in the northeastern, mid-Atlantic, and midwestern states, where the wide variety of religions and ethnic groups were able to amass the necessary capital to fund hospitals in the late nineteenth and early twentieth centuries.[27]

ORGANIZATION AND FUNCTIONS OF HOSPITALS

Hospitals differ from each other and from other institutions, not only by their ownership and control but also according to the functions that they perform. Four of the functions—patient care, health promotion, biomedical research, and education—replicate the broad functions of the U.S. health care system, as shown in Table 1–1. The fifth function, administration, is not unique to hospitals but is a requisite function of all institutions. It is important to understand all of these functions and their recordkeeping implications in terms of the distinctions between hospitals and businesses.

American hospitals are similar to businesses and have become more so since the passage of Medicare and Medicaid legislation in 1965, which created a large base of paying population for which hospitals competed. Since the mid-1960s, nonprofit hospitals have been forced to adopt some of the management activities, such as marketing, employed by for-profit hospitals.[28] It is not uncommon for nonprofit hospitals today to have marketing managers or marketing departments. Nonprofit hospitals were again forced to adopt some of their for-profit counterparts' strategies in 1983 when the federal government changed its method of Medicare reimbursement from "reasonable cost" to a fixed rate based on the patient's diagnosis.[29] Thus, all hospitals were forced to become more efficient or lose money when treating Medicare patients.

Several important differences also set hospitals apart from businesses. The major difference, and probably the one that has the most effect on records creation, is the nature of the hospital's organizational structure. Hospital organization is not strictly hierarchical but comprises two main components: an administrative component and a clinical or medical component. Each component is organized differently, and no theoretical model integrates them.[30]

The administrative component, which is responsible for hospital management, is usually organized in a strict hierarchical fashion. The organization of the medical component, which is responsible for patient care, education, and biomedical research, is flatter, and its members typically work in teams across departmental lines. To complicate matters further, the two components overlap, and many hospital employees report to two supervisors, an administrator and a physician. The chief technician of a pathology laboratory, for example, generally reports to the physician in charge of the medical operations of the laboratory and to the administrator responsible for the laboratory's financial operations. Many hospitals have a joint committee in place to bridge the gap between the medical and administrative components. This administrative/medical dichotomy, which is referred to in the professional literature as a "dual authority structure," has also affected the credentials of hospital chief executive officers, which seem to alternate between management and medical degrees. The current trend in nonprofit hospitals is toward physician chief executive officers.[31]

Another significant difference between hospitals and businesses is that while businesses employ all the individuals on their staffs, physicians who work in hospitals may not be employed by the hospital. In the past, very few physicians were paid by hospitals; instead, hospitals extended privileges to physicians to admit their patients. The patient paid two fees, one to the physician and the other to the hospital for use of the facilities, nursing care, diagnostic tests, medical supplies, and medication. In contrast, certain types of physician, such as radiologists and anesthesiologists, have traditionally been employed by hospitals and receive a salary. Different arrangements between physicians and hospitals are now common practice, and hospitals routinely employ physicians individually or as groups. Newer alliances between hospitals and groups of physicians, called physician hospital organizations, are the result of pressures to contain costs. Their main purpose is to contract with managed care organizations (HMOs and preferred provider organizations) and self-insured employers, and to manage health care delivery. To further complicate the issue, physicians in teaching hospitals may also have an appointment at an affiliated medical school. Whatever the arrangement between physicians and hospitals, a two-pronged organizational scheme is the prevailing pattern.

There are several significant differences between hospital patients and consumers of business products and services. Patients are not always able to comparison shop; they generally are not concerned with the cost of health care, especially if they have health insurance; and they have little control over what they are buying because the physician decides which drug or procedure is best for them (although sometimes patients will be offered a choice among a small number of treatment options).

Other differences between hospitals and businesses include the fact that hospitals do not manufacture a uniform product or provide a uniform service; rather, hospitals provide health care services that are tailored to each patient. In addition, physicians significantly influence both the supply and the demand for a service or product, whereas in business supply and demand are determined independently. Finally, in business technological advances are usually cost-efficient; in hospitals they are usually not, since technological advances increase cost because specially trained personnel are needed to operate new and often expensive diagnostic and therapeutic equipment.[32] There may, however, be several departments or services within a hospital that are run as businesses. Hospital pharmacies, gift shops (often run by the auxiliary), and optical shops are examples. In addition, a hospital's parent company may own for-profit businesses, such as nursing homes, alcohol and drug treatment centers, freestanding emergency centers, ambulance services, HMOs, doctors' office buildings, progressive care retirement communities, hotels, and parking facilities.

Hospital Organization   The clinical activities of hospitals are usually organized into medical departments or services, but there is no standard organizational model. One of three criteria is generally used in defining departments: (1) the organ or organ system that is treated, (2) the skill involved, and (3) the age or sex of the patients. The number of medical departments in a hospital varies according to the hospital's size and degree of specialization, but most general hospitals include the following departments: anesthesiology, emergency medicine, internal medicine, obstetrics/gynecology, pathology, pediatrics, psychiatry/neurology, radiology/

diagnostic imaging, and surgery. More specialized medical departments include ophthalmology, preventive medicine, and urology.[33]

The nonclinical activities of hospitals fall into six categories: governance, external relations, fiscal affairs, operations management, facilities management, and human resources. Hospitals are often organized so that vice presidents are responsible for these activities.

The following sections, organized by hospital function, discuss the activities and mechanisms peculiar to hospitals, which archivists need to understand to make sense of the resulting records.

Administration   All institutions engage in administrative activities that are necessary to conduct business. Hospitals are no exception; they engage in activities related, for example, to institutional governance, fiscal management, personnel management, and research management, much as other businesses do. Two hospital activities, however, accreditation and regulation, warrant further discussion because they are complex and distinctive.

Since 1952, hospital *accreditation* has been carried out by the Joint Commission on Accreditation of Healthcare Organizations (JCAHO). Representatives of five organizations make up the commission: the American College of Physicians, the American College of Surgeons, the American Dental Association, the American Hospital Association, and the American Medical Association. In accrediting hospitals, the JCAHO is concerned with three areas: (1) quality of patient care, (2) hospital organization and administration, and (3) hospital facilities. The accreditation process consists of an extensive survey that is filled out by hospital administrators and a site visit by a JCAHO accreditation team consisting of a physician, one or two nurses, and sometimes a hospital administrator. Hospitals may be accredited for three years with or without contingencies, and hospitals that are regarded as "marginal" are publicly identified as such. Beginning in mid-1993, the JCAHO instituted unannounced surveys of randomly selected accredited organizations to better gauge and ensure compliance with commission standards. The surveys are conducted at the midaccreditation point of a 5 percent sample of all organizations that participate in the three-year accreditation process. One surveyor will conduct a one-day survey limited to the five performance areas in which hospitals generally have the most problems: safety management, life safety, medical staff appointment and privileging, infection control, and governance. In 1995, the JCAHO will implement new standards that are organized functionally instead of departmentally. Although the JCAHO is a private organization and JCAHO accreditation is not mandated by law, Medicare and Medicaid legislation requires hospitals to meet standards equal to JCAHO standards to receive payment; thus, virtually all hospitals seek JCAHO accreditation.

Hospitals are the most extensively regulated institution in the United States.[34] Since the passage of Medicare and Medicaid legislation, hospital *regulation* has increased dramatically. Before that time, regulations were aimed mostly at the condition of the facility. Today, they have been expanded to cover the quality and cost of care. Regulation of hospitals has been described as lacking in "consistency, parsimony and clarity."[35] This is because hospitals are regulated by a wide range of private organizations (e.g., Blue Cross and the JCAHO) and public agencies representing all three levels of government, without any attempt at coordination. Often, the regulations of different bodies conflict with one another.

Hospital regulation falls into four categories: (1) facilities regulation, (2) planning regulation, (3) quality and appropriateness of care, and (4) payment.[36] All states require hospitals to be licensed, although the scope of mandatory *facilities regulation* varies from state to state, and in some states JCAHO accreditation guarantees state licensure. State licensing regulations usually concern hospital organization (requiring an organized governing body, organized medical staff, and administrator), the provision of certain specified services, and standards for facilities, equipment, and personnel. State governments also have certain building code requirements that apply to all facilities. These include regulations regarding elevator and boiler performance, waste disposal, fire safety, and electrical and plumbing facilities. In addition, hospitals are subject to state and federal legislation that affects, for example, the dispensing of narcotics and alcohol, the disposal of hazardous waste, radiation safety, water and air quality, labor practices (including job safety), and educational requirements for teaching programs.

Planning is defined by the American Hospital Association as "an orderly process for determining the health care needs of a specific population and developing an appropriate health care capability to meet those needs."[37] The federal government was involved in hospital *planning regulation* from 1946, when the Hill-Burton Hospital Survey and Construction Act was passed, until 1986. This legislation provided for hospital construction or renovation mostly in rural areas where there was a shortage of beds. Currently, some states control capital expenditures for construction, expansion, and modernization of health care facilities as well as the purchase of costly technology, such as radiologic imaging devices. The purpose of this legislation is to avoid unnecessary duplication of services and to control costs. This certificate-of-need review process involves considerable documentation and lengthy reviews at the local, regional, and state levels.

The quality and appropriateness of care, the third type of hospital regulation, has been in effect since the passage of the 1965 Medicare legislation, which requires that the appropriateness and necessity of care provided to Medicare patients be evaluated by an examination of patient records. Because of this regulation, hospitals established quality assurance and utilization review committees to monitor and analyze patient admissions, length of stay, and allocation of resources. In 1972 the federal government legislated the creation of professional standards review organizations (PSROs) comprised of local physicians who were paid by the DHHS to monitor physician behavior and evaluate the quality and necessity of services covered by Medicare and Medicaid. Since 1984, the review contracts have been awarded to peer review organizations (PROs), which are nonprofit, community based, physician-directed agencies and have more authority than the PSROs. One PRO per state reviews admissions and re-admissions, validates diagnoses, and reviews exceptional cases and quality of care. Each PRO has a contract with the Health Care Financing

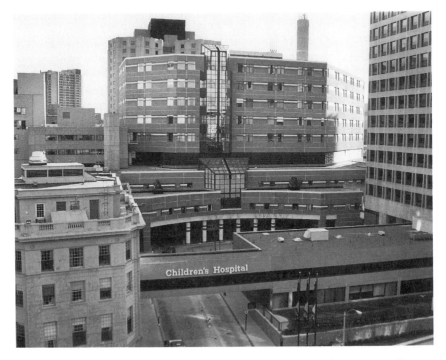

FIGURE 2–2 Children's Hospital, Boston, 1990. A corner of the Hunnewell Building is visible on the left. The thirteen-floor John F. Enders Pediatric Research Building is located to the far right. *Source:* Children's Hospital Archives

Administration that specifies how it will carry out these activities. If medical audits reveal unacceptable practice, the government does not reimburse the offending hospital for Medicare patients. In many cases hospitals participate in the review process through in-house professional services review departments, which are monitored by the PRO.

The quality of care in hospitals is also regulated by several obligatory committees that seek to ensure a high standard of patient care. These committees are generally overseen by a hospital's Professional Services Review Committee or another group with responsibilities for quality assurance. They include the Credentials Committee (which ensures that physicians have the necessary and appropriate credentials), the Infection Control Committee, the Medical Records Committee (which reviews the "content, appropriateness and timeliness"[38] of official patient records), the Pharmacy and Therapeutics Committee (which reviews drug utilization and patient responses), the Radiation Committee, the Safety Committee, and the Tissue Committee (which examines tissue removed from patients to determine whether surgery was indeed necessary).

Whereas the other types of regulation indirectly aim at controlling costs, the final type of hospital regulation, *regulation of payment,* directly influences the cost of hospital services. At both state and local levels, retrospective reimbursement has been replaced by prospective payment. At the state level, payment regulation is sometimes controlled by a rate-setting commission that prospectively approves rates for hospital services. The federal government controls rates for in-patient hospital care to Medicare and Medicaid patients through diagnosis-related groups (DRGs). Historically, only fees for hospital services were regulated; physicians were reimbursed according to a system of "customary, prevailing, and reasonable" charges. This changed with the adoption by federal regulators, some private insurers, and other third-party payers of the recently formulated resource-based relative value scale (RBRVS) for physician fees. Developed at the Harvard School of Public Health, the RBRVS standardizes physician fees according to three factors: (1) the duration and intensity of the work, (2) the cost of providing the service, and (3) the cost of physician training.[39]

Just as hospitals are accredited by the JCAHO and licensed by the states, health care practitioners are also licensed.[40] Licensure usually involves fulfilling certain educational requirements and passing an examination. Which of the numerous health care professions require licensure, however, varies among the states. In most states the hospital is responsible for ensuring that medical and technical personnel meet governmental standards; therefore, hospitals often employ registrars whose function is to document the credentials of physicians and other health care practitioners. (See Chapter 5 for more information on licensing health care professionals.)

Patient Care Patient care, which encompasses diagnosis and treatment, is the primary function of hospitals and what distinguishes them from other institutions within and outside of the health care system. Patient care is often divided into three levels—primary care, secondary care, and tertiary care—based on the severity of the condition to be treated. Primary care denotes care that is simple to give, or the evaluation of a condition and referral to a specialist. Although primary care does not require hospitalization, individuals may receive primary care in a hospital setting. Treating individuals with infections, or victims of minor accidents, and providing annual physical examinations are examples of primary care. Secondary care is more specialized care for conditions that require day surgery or hospitalization. Treating victims of burns or serious accidents and extracting tonsils are examples of secondary care. Tertiary care is the most specialized level of care and generally involves the most advanced medical knowledge and technology available. Because of this, most teaching hospitals that are part of academic health centers specialize in tertiary care. Tertiary care includes treatment for cancer and for congenital and metabolic disorders.[41] Some hospitals engage in all three levels of care, although many smaller hospitals refer tertiary care cases to larger hospitals.

Diagnoses may be made by health care professionals without the aid of technology (as when they prescribe treatment on the basis of their observations or information provided by patients) or with the aid of technology. There are three main catories of diagnostic technology: sample analysis, intrinsic energy analysis, and external energy probes. Sample analysis consists of analyzing the chemical and cellular components of body fluids and tissues. Examples of sample analysis include blood tests, tumor biopsies, and spectroscopy. Intrinsic energy analysis measures internal energy conditions, such as temperature, sound, and pulse. Electroencephalographs, for example, are devices that record the electrical activity of the brain. The third category of diagnostic technology, external energy probes, is used to determine the size, shape, and location of internal organs. External energy probes work by directing beams of energy into the patient and analyzing the energy that comes out. Examples of external energy probes are ultrasound and x-ray imagers.[42]

Hospital laboratories are an important element in patient diagnosis. Two types of laboratory—clinical pathology and research—may exist in a hospital, but only clinical pathology laboratories are involved with diagnosis. Through sample analysis, they provide information that assists health care personnel in diagnosing disease.

Patient treatment may be classified as internal therapy (medication), external therapy (casts, bandages, advice on life-style changes), mental therapy, or surgery. Patient treatment may further be distinguished according to whether the patient remains in the hospital overnight (inpatient) or is treated and released (outpatient). Hospital outpatient departments first appeared in the 1920s, and since then they have increased in number, scope, and complexity.[43] Outpatient services consist of emergency care and general diagnosis and treatment for nonemergency conditions to individuals referred by themselves or a physician. It is noteworthy that in the last several years the length of hospital stays has decreased, and some procedures, such as cataract surgery, that were previously performed on an in-patient basis are now performed as ambulatory surgery, eliminating the need for an overnight hospital stay. This change is due to improved techniques and to revised Medicare and Medicaid reimbursement regulations aimed at cost containment.

Advances in communications technology have significantly altered the delivery of patient care. Computer networks link physicians to one another and physicians' homes and offices to hospital laboratories and finance departments. Physicians can readily update medical records using voice recognition technology, and diagnostic imaging departments are able to store images on optical disks instead of film. Furthermore, patients can carry with them their medical record on a card about the size of a credit card. For an overview of how computerization has affected health care, see Nina W. Matheson, "Computerization and a New Era for Archives" in Nancy McCall and Lisa A. Mix, eds., *Designing Archival Programs in the Health Fields* (Baltimore: Johns Hopkins University Press, 1994).

Health Promotion   Health promotion, also called consumer health education, is the process of communication and education that "helps each individual to learn how to achieve and maintain a reasonable level of health appropriate to his particular needs and interests, and to be motivated to follow health . . . practices which contribute to his state of health and well-being."[44] Historically, hospitals in the United States have not participated very actively in health promotion. This trend seems to be reversing due to the need to contain costs: by 1987, health promotion programs were offered in more than one third of U.S. hospitals.[45] Community hospitals are especially conscientious about health promotion programs, and it is not unusual for them to offer (free or at a moderate cost) literature concerning health issues and health education classes in how to stop smoking, reduce stress, or maintain a healthier diet. Health promotion programs may also include health support groups, health screening, physical fitness classes, family life education, and rehabilitation.

Biomedical Research   Biomedical research is similar to scientific/technological research, with the exception that biomedical research may be more clinical; therefore, the records of research done in hospitals are often similar to those produced by research in a university.[46] Hospitals may embark on research projects jointly with universities or corporations, thus affecting the location and ownership of project records. Biomedical research in the hospital setting may be scientific/technological in nature or a combination of scientific/technological and medical. Recently, the trend in hospitals has been to increase research and development activities to produce new products with commercial potential. Often these activities are conducted in cooperation with pharmaceutical companies. This type of diversification is aimed at enabling hospitals to remain viable in a competitive environment.[47]

Biomedical research in whatever setting is regulated just as scientific/ technological research is regulated. Hospitals, like other institutions performing research involving animals or humans, must have animal care committees and human subject committees. These are federally mandated committees that closely monitor federally funded research involving animals or humans. If abuses occur, committee members are obliged to report them to the National Institutes of Health. (For more information on biomedical research and biomedical research facilities, see Chapter 4.)

Education   In a hospital setting, education and training may occur at many levels. Hospital personnel are given on-the-job training in infection control and safety procedures; laboratory and radiology technicians are trained; nursing students are provided with undergraduate education or specialty training; graduate students earn master's degrees in nursing, dietetics, or physical therapy; other graduate students work on research projects in hospital departments or laboratories as part of doctoral degree work; medical students go through rotations, which lead to M.D. degrees; physicians are given postgraduate education as residents or fellows; and allied health care professionals in all disciplines attend hospital-sponsored in-service programs or continuing education courses to retain their certification or licensure or to update their knowledge and skills. To this end it is not uncommon for hospitals to have an education department, or for medical departments to hire managers to deal primarily with education. Hospitals may also provide the clinical facilities necessary for programs that they do not sponsor. In addition, hospitals often provide trustee education and management development courses. (See Chapter 5 for information on educational institutions and programs for health care– related occupations.)

Certain hospitals are identified as teaching hospitals. According to the

American Hospital Association, a teaching hospital is "a hospital that allocates a substantial part of its resources to conduct, in its own name or in formal association with a college, courses of instruction in the health disciplines that lead to the granting of recognized certificates, diplomas, or degrees, or that are required for professional certification or licensure."[48] Although this definition does not mention research, the reality is that the majority of teaching hospitals also engage in biomedical research, and hospitals that engage in research are also usually defined as teaching hospitals.

Historically, the majority of teaching hospitals in the United States were public hospitals; today, however, the majority of teaching hopitals are voluntary.[49] For-profit hospitals generally avoid engaging in teaching and biomedical research because they are not profitable activities; however, a few investor-owned companies began purchasing or leasing teaching hospitals in the early 1980s, for a variety of complex reasons.[50] In 1991, 19 percent (1,238) of all hospitals were teaching hospitals. Of these, 30 percent were government owned (18 percent state and local, 12 percent federal) and 70 percent were privately owned (67 percent not-for-profit, 3 percent for-profit). Although the term "teaching hospital" traditionally referred to affiliation with a medical school, today it also denotes affiliation with other educational institutions. The Veterans Administration Hospital in Ann Arbor, Michigan, for example, is affiliated with the University of Michigan Medical School and thirty-four other educational institutions.

NURSING HOMES

Nursing homes and hospitals are similar in many respects. For example, they both provide in-patient medical care, are heavily regulated, are licensed by the JCAHO, and provide training for health care professionals. Yet they have one basic difference: nursing homes are primarily places where people live and secondarily where they receive medical care. For this reason health care professionals play a less significant role in controlling and operating nursing homes.[51]

Until relatively recently, hospitals provided long-term health care for elderly and convalescent people. Although hospitals still provide long-term care, nursing homes provide most of it. In fact, the nursing home industry is the third largest element of the health care system.[52] In 1991 there were 15,913 certified nursing homes in the United States,[53] and $59.9 billion (about 7.5 percent of the total spent on health care) was spent on nursing home care.[54]

Most likely the first nursing home began in the early 1930s in Chicago or Detroit.[55] The Social Security Act of 1935 increased the number of people who were able to purchase nursing home care and caused proprietary nursing homes to dominate the market. Until World War II, nursing homes generally were small, run by the owner, and staffed by the immediate family. With increasing governmental regulation of the industry, especially Social Security Act amendments in 1950, 1972, and 1974, these "mom and pop" nursing homes were forced out of business because they could not afford to comply. Nevertheless, proprietary nursing homes are still the norm. Since the late 1960s, publicly held corporations have owned and operated nursing homes, and in 1991 for-profit organizations owned 67.3 percent of the nursing homes in the United States, while 25.9 percent were owned by nonprofit organizations and 6.8 percent by government.[56]

Until 1989 nursing homes were licensed to provide two types of care: skilled care and intermediate care. Skilled care provided services that "(1) require the skills of technical or professional personnel . . . [and] (2) are provided either directly by or under the supervision . . . of such personnel."[57] Intermediate care consisted of "health-related care and services to individuals who do not require the degree of care and treatment which a hospital or skilled nursing facility is designed to provide, but who . . . require care and services (above the level of room and board) which can be made available to them only through institutional facilities."[58] Nursing homes were designated either as skilled nursing facilities, which the federal government reimbursed under Medicare and Medicaid, or as intermediate care facilities, which were reimbursed under Medicaid only; or they provided both levels of care. Since 1990, all nursing homes are referred to as nursing facilities and are required to provide the same level of care.

Nursing homes engage in four of the five functions in which hospitals engage: administration, patient care, health promotion, and education and training. The most important function, patient care, includes nursing and medical care (e.g., injections, catheterizations, and physical therapy), personal care (assistance in eating, dressing, and bathing), and residential services (food preparation, cleaning, and organizing social activities).

For skilled nursing facilities to participate in Medicare and Medicaid, they must provide or provide for the following services: nursing, dietetic, specialized rehabilitative, pharmaceutical, laboratory, radiologic, dental, and social. They are also required to keep medical records, have infection control and utilization review committees, provide activities for nursing home residents, meet local health and safety standards, have a transfer agreement with a hospital, and meet disaster preparedness requirements.[59]

HOSPICES

Hospice is a term used to identify both institutions and programs. The National Hospice Organization defines a hospice as "a centrally administered program of palliative and support services which provides physical, psychological, social, and spiritual care for dying persons and their families. Services are provided by a medically supervised interdisciplinary team of professionals and volunteers. Hospice services are available in both the home and inpatient settings. . . . Bereavement services are available to the family."[60] This definition covers the five basic elements of hospice care: (1) patient and family are treated as a unit, (2) care—consisting at a minimum of medical direction, nursing services, social services, spiritual support, volunteer services, and bereavement counseling—is managed by an interdisciplinary team, (3) patient care is palliative rather than curative, (4) care is available in the patient's home, and (5) bereavement care is provided for the family after the patient's death.[61]

In the past, "hospice" referred to inns run by religious orders. The first health care–related hospice opened in London in 1967 under the direction of Dame Cicely Saunders. The first hospice in the United States was the Hospice of Connecticut, in New Haven, which opened in 1974, and by 1992 the number of hospice programs had grown to about 2,000.[62] The hospice concept caught on in part because the roles of hospitals and nursing homes changed with the increase in governmental regulation of their utilization and because the federal government no longer viewed them as the most appropriate (i.e., cost effective) institutions to deal with terminally ill patients (those with less than six months to live). In 1983 federal laws that allow Medicare reimbursement for home hospice care went into effect.

Just as there is a variety of types of hospital, so is there a range of types of hospice. The ownership of hospices may be private and for-profit, voluntary, or governmental. Hospices may be independent or part of larger institutions such as hospitals, skilled nursing facilities, HMOs, home health agencies, or psychiatric facilities. In addition, there are several models for hospices owned by hospitals. They may be freestanding institutions, a discrete unit within the hospital, or beds scattered throughout the hospital. Community-based hospice programs usually do not provide direct care. Instead, they coordinate care by contracting for services from existing agencies and hospitals. In 1992 26 percent of hospices were divisions of hospitals, 41 percent were owned by independent corporations, and 20 percent were affiliated with home health agencies.[63]

Hospices perform four of the five functions of a hospital: administration, patient care, education, and biomedical research activities. Hospices have little involvement in health promotion because of the nature of the patient clientele, although services to families might be classified under this heading. Educational activities in a hospice may include the training of residents and interns if the hospice is connected to a teaching hospital; otherwise these activities are limited to the hospice staff, who most likely did not receive training or education specific to hospices before working in one. Although hospices seem unlikely settings for research, some of them engage, for example, in studies of approaches to palliative care or antitumor therapies.[64]

Because hospices are a relatively recent development in the health care system, their regulation by the government did not become an issue until the 1980s. In 1983 the JCAHO and the National Hospice Organization developed standards for evaluating hospice programs. Also, Blue Cross/Blue Shield, Medicare, and Medicaid reimburse providers for certain hospice services.

AMBULATORY CARE SETTINGS

Ambulatory care is generally provided in one of two settings, physician offices or clinics.[65] Although most ambulatory care is provided by physicians in office-based practices, it is also common for individuals to go directly to a hospital clinic for primary care, often because they do not have health insurance.[66] *Physician offices* may be organized as individual or group practices, although the number of solo practices is declining as the number and size of group practices increase.[67] Solo practitioners are most often specialists who provide secondary care only. Physicians may also contract their services out on a part-time basis or may be part of an independent practice plan or association, in which they contract with a prepaid group health plan but see patients in their own offices.

The term *group practice* refers to a variety of legal and financial arrangements. Legal arrangements include sole proprietorships, associations, professional corporations, and partnerships. Financial arrangements most commonly include situations in which the patient pays and the physician is remunerated on a fee-for-service basis, or the patient prepays and the physician is either remunerated at a flat rate for each patient or on salary.[68] A growing trend is hospital-based group practices. This may mean that the group of physicians comprises the hospital's medical staff; alternatively, the group and hospital may be independent, and, while the group treats all of its in-patients in the affiliated hospital, the hospital also accepts patients from other physicians. The first group medical practice was organized in 1887 in Minnesota by Dr. William W.

Mayo, who formed a partnership with his two sons. Today the trend is away from solo practice and toward group practices, which may be devoted to the practice of general or family medicine, a single specialty (such as ophthalmology or obstetrics and gynecology), or multiple specialties.[69]

Until the early part of the twentieth century, the term *clinic* connoted medical charity. Today a clinic is usually defined as a setting in which diagnostic or therapeutic services are provided on an ambulatory basis rather than to in-patients.[70] Clinics are numerous and varied. They may be general or specialized, and freestanding or part of a larger institution. (See Table 2–2 for a categorization of clinic types according to the clientele served and the condition diagnosed or treated.) Non-institutionally based clinics may be sponsored by private individuals or corporations (e.g., American Medical International Diagnostic Services); local, state, or national government (East Boston Neighborhood Health Center); voluntary entities (the American Cancer Society's cancer detection clinics); or a combination of these groups. Freestanding ambulatory care facilities providing emergency and urgent care services were first established in 1973 in Delaware and Rhode Island.

Institutionally based clinics are found in institutions whose primary function is health care related as well as in those whose primary function is not health care related. Institutions such as HMOs, holistic or alternative health centers, and hospitals (emergency services, ambulatory services, and satellite clinics) are in the first category. Business and industry (employee health clinics and wellness programs), prisons, private homes (home care[71] programs sponsored by hospitals, visiting nurse associations, public health agencies, and health care companies),[72] and schools are in the second category.

ARCHIVES PROGRAMS IN HEALTH CARE DELIVERY FACILITIES

HOSPITALS

Although some hospitals and academic health centers have active archival programs, the percentage is small. The Society of American Archivists' 1991 directory lists only twenty hospital archivists; the New England Archivists' 1991 handbook and directory lists an additional three hospital archivists; the *Guide to Repositories of the Science, Technology and Health Care Round Table*[73] mentions another twelve archival programs collecting hospital records. (The archives program at Children's Hospital, Boston, is too new to have been listed in any of these directories.) The American Hospital Association's *Guide to Historical Collections in Hospital and Healthcare*

Administration adds about 250 institutions (including state universities) to the number collecting hospital records, but most of these institutions do not have programs run by professional archivists. Although these numbers do not include city and state archives that collect hospital records, they still indicate that only a small percentage (somewhere in the neighborhood of 5 percent) of hospitals have programs to preserve their historical records.

A cursory search of Research Libraries Information Network on-line data base (RLIN) provided more evidence that hospitals are underdocumented. A corporate heading search of "hospitals" uncovered 2,250 entries; the same type of search for "colleges and universities" yielded 21,000 entries. Even if one takes into account the fact that academic institutions are more likely than freestanding hospitals to have listed their records in RLIN, there are approximately ten times as many entries for colleges and universities than for hospitals.

HOSPICES AND NURSING HOMES

If hospitals are underdocumented, hospices and nursing homes are virtually undocumented. In searching the various guides to archival repositories, I did not find a single hospice or nursing home that had its own archives program. A search of RLIN yielded no entries for hospices and only 59 for nursing homes.

It is unlikely that health care facilities other than hospitals will choose to maintain in-house archival programs. Perhaps the most reasonable way to document nursing homes, hospices, and ambulatory clinics is to identify selected records to be placed with a city or state archives, historical society, or other appropriate repository.

Although the data presented here are more impressionistic than scientific, they clearly demonstrate that health care delivery facilities are in need of systematic documentation. I am not advocating that all health care delivery facilities maintain in-house archival programs that document in detail their every aspect. I do believe that these institutions should consider developing archival programs (in-house or external) to suit their specific needs and capabilities. The purpose of this work is to facilitate development of such programs.

NOTES

1. Lois Rakus Keefe, "A Conceptual Model of Ambulatory Care Programs and Delivery Systems in the U.S." (unpublished thesis in partial fulfillment of the

requirements for fellowship in the American College of Hospital
Administrators, Chicago, December 1981), 15.

2. Morris J. Vogel, review of *The Care of Strangers: The Rise of America's Hospital System*, by Charles E. Rosenberg, *Bulletin of the History of Medicine* 62 (Summer 1988): 284.

3. American Hospital Association, *Hospital Statistics, 1992–93 Edition* (Chicago: American Hospital Association, 1992). The statistics in this publication are based on 1991 figures. Unless otherwise noted, all subsequent statistics are from this source.

4. The editors of *The Chronicle of Higher Education, The Almanac of Higher Education* (Chicago: University of Chicago Press, 1991).

5. Katharine R. Levit et al., "National Health Expenditures 1990," *Health Care Financing Review* 13, no. 1 (1991): 29–54.

6. Stephen J. Williams and Paul R. Torrens, eds., *Introduction to Health Services* (New York: John Wiley & Sons, 1984), 172.

7. *American Hospital Association Guide to the Health Care Field, 1987 Edition* (Chicago: American Hospital Association, 1987), A13.

8. Anthony R. Kovner, and contributors, *Health Care Delivery in the United States* 4th ed. (New York: Springer Publishing Company, 1990), 305.

9. The Clinical Center provides patient care only to individuals with illnesses that are being studied at one of the institutes; general diagnostic, treatment, and emergency services are not offered.

10. J. Rogers Hollingsworth, *A Political Economy of Medicine: Great Britain and the United States* (Baltimore: Johns Hopkins University Press, 1986), 80–81.

11. Ibid., 5.

12. Ibid., 75.

13. It is interesting to note that Jewish hospitals fall into the last category rather than the first, for they are supported by members of the Jewish community but are not controlled by the synagogue. Similarly, black hospitals are community hospitals supported by the African-American community.

14. Revised and updated from Florence A. Wilson and Duncan Newhauser, *Health Services in the United States* (Cambridge, Mass.: Ballinger, 1985), 9.

15. Hollingsworth, *Political Economy of Medicine*, 74.

16. J. Rogers Hollingsworth and Ellen Jane Hollingsworth, *Controversy about American Hospitals: Funding, Ownership, and Performance* (Washington, D.C.: American Enterprise Institute for Public Policy Research, 1987), 63.

17. Ekaterini Siafaca, *Investor-Owned Hospitals and Their Role in the Changing U.S. Health Care System* (New York: F & S Press, 1981), 117.

18. Russell C. Coile, Jr., *The New Medicine: Reshaping Medical Practice and Health Care Management* (Rockville, Md.: Aspen Publishers, 1990), 29.

19. Most health maintenance organizations do not own hospitals but have agreements with specific hospitals where their members are treated.

20. National Medical Enterprises, Inc., Annual Report, 1992.

21. "The Hospital World's Hard-Driving Money Man," *New York Times*, 5 Oct. 1993, D1.

22. Kovner, *Health Care Delivery*, 143.
23. Paul Starr, *The Social Transformation of American Medicine: The Rise of a Sovereign Profession and the Making of a Vast Industry* (New York: Basic Books, 1982), 202.
24. "Frustrated Firms Open Their Own Clinics to Try to Control Workers' Medical Costs," *Wall Street Journal*, 23 March 1993, B1.
25. Siafaca, *Investor-Owned Hospitals*, 62.
26. Hollingsworth and Hollingsworth, *Controversy about American Hospitals*, 27, 62.
27. Ibid., 26–27.
28. Donald W. Light, "Corporate Medicine for Profit," *Scientific American* 255 (December 1986):42.
29. Diagnosis-related groups (DRGs) are a form of prospective payment under Medicare for in-patient hospital services. Under this system, hospitals are paid a specified amount for services provided based on a patient's classification into one of approximately 500 DRGs, regardless of what the care actually costs and with some adjustments made for teaching hospitals and regional variations in cost of living. Psychiatric, rehabilitation, children's, and long-term hospitals are excluded from DRG regulations.
30. Luther P. Christman and Michael A. Counte, *Hospital Organization and Health Care Delivery* (Boulder: Westview Press, 1981), 28.
31. Coile, *The New Medicine*, 242.
32. Jonathon S. Rakich and Kurt Darr, eds., *Hospital Organization and Management: Text and Readings* (New York: SP Medical and Scientific Books, 1983), 597–600.
33. Kovner, *Health Care Delivery*, 161–62.
34. Siafaca, *Investor-Owned Hospitals*, 29.
35. American Hospital Association, *Hospital Regulation: Report of the Special Committee on the Regulatory Process* (Chicago: American Hospital Association, 1977), 2.
36. Siafaca, *Investor-Owned Hospitals*, 33, and American Hospital Association, *Hospital Regulation* (1977), 113.
37. American Hospital Association, *Hospital Regulation* (1977), 11.
38. Donald I. Snook, Jr., and Edita M. Kaye, *A Guide to Health Care Joint Ventures* (Rockville, Md.: Aspen Publishers, 1987), 195.
39. William C. Hsiao et al., "Resource-Based Relative Values: An Overview," *Journal of the American Medical Association* 260 (October 1988): 2347–53.
40. The American Hospital Association defines licensure as "the process by which an agency of government grants permission to an individual to engage in a given occupation, upon finding that the applicant has attained the minimal degree of competency necessary to ensure that the public health, safety, and welfare be reasonably well protected." American Hospital Association, *Guidelines: Licensure of Health Care Personnel* (Chicago: American Hospital Association, 1977), 1.
41. James M. Rosser and Howard E. Mossberg, *An Analysis of Health Care Delivery* (New York: John Wiley & Sons, 1977), 16.
42. Williams and Torrens, *Health Services*, 287.

43. Milton I. Roemer, *Ambulatory Health Services* (Rockville, Md: Aspen Publishers, 1981), 48.
44. Myra E. Madnick, *Consumer Health Education: A Guide to Hospital-Based Programs* (Wakefield, Mass.: Nursing Resources, 1980), 1.
45. Coile, *The New Medicine*, 152.
46. For a discussion of scientific/technological research from the standpoint of its component activities, see Joan K(rizack) Haas et al., *Appraising the Records of Modern Science and Technology: A Guide* (Cambridge: MIT, 1985).
47. Coile, *The New Medicine*, 35.
48. "Definition of a Teaching Hospital," American Hospital Association Memorandum, 11–15 Nov. 1967, as quoted in William E. Hassam, *Hospital Pharmacy* (Philadelphia: Lea & Febiger, 1986), 45.
49. Hollingsworth and Hollingsworth, *Controversy about American Hospitals*, 47.
50. Committee on Implications of For-Profit Enterprise in Health Care, Institute of Medicine, Bradford H. Gray, ed., *For-Profit Enterprise in Health Care* (Washington, D.C.: National Academy Press, 1986), 145.
51. Catherine Hawes and Charles D. Phillips, "The Changing Structure of the Nursing Home Industry and the Impact of Ownership on Quality, Cost and Access," in Gray, ed., *For-Profit Enterprise*, 492–541.
52. Ibid., 492.
53. American Health Care Association, *Issue and Data Book for Long Term Care* (Washington, D.C.: American Health Care Association, 1993), 49.
54. "Aid for Chronic Illness and Other Long-Term Care," *New York Times*, 21 Feb. 1993, L25.
55. Wesley Wiley Rogers, *General Administration in the Nursing Home* (Boston: CBI, 1980), 166.
56. American Health Care Association, *Issues and Data Book*, 49.
57. From the *Code of Federal Regulations* as quoted in Bruce C. Vladek, *Unloving Care: The Nursing Home Tragedy* (New York: Basic Books, 1980), 135.
58. Idem.
59. *Federal Register*, 39, no. 12, pt. III (Thursday, 17 Jan. 1974): 2238–49.
60. National Hospice Organization, *Standards of a Hospice Program of Care*, 6th rev. (McLean, Va.: National Hospice Organization, 1979).
61. Paul R. Torrens, ed., *Hospice Programs and Public Policy* (Chicago: American Hospital Association, 1985), 7, 37.
62. Telephone conversation with Glenn Gillen, Communications Manager for the National Hospice Organization, 28 June 1993.
63. Idem.
64. Jack M. Zimmerman, *Hospice: Complete Care for the Terminally Ill* (Baltimore: Urban and Schwarzenberg, 1986), 46.
65. A case could be made that pharmacies and health food stores, where pharmacists and employees advise customers on over-the-counter medications, vitamin therapy, and homeopathic remedies, are also settings for ambulatory care.
66. Williams and Torrens, *Health Services*, 139, 156.

67. Coile, *The New Medicine*, 240.
68. Steven Jonas, *Health Care Delivery in the United States* (New York: Springer Publishing Company, 1981), 146.
69. Milton I. Roemer, *An Introduction to the U.S. Health Care System* (New York: Springer Publishing Company, 1986), 21–22.
70. Roemer, *Ambulatory Health Services*, 29.
71. Home care is defined by the Joint Commission on Accreditation of Healthcare Organizations as providing professional nursing and at least one other therapeutic service. See JCAHO, *Accreditation Manual for Hospitals, 1988* (Chicago: JCAHO, 1987), 53.
72. The bulk of the records documenting home care resides with the provider of care and not in patients' homes.
73. This guide was produced by the Science, Technology and Health Care Round Table of the Society of American Archivists in 1988.

SELECTED ANNOTATED BIBLIOGRAPHY

Three outstanding books on the history of hospitals in the United States are Charles E. Rosenberg, *The Care of Strangers: The Rise of America's Hospital System* (New York: Basic Books, 1987), which discusses hospitals in their social context from 1800 to 1920; Rosemary Stevens, *In Sickness and Wealth: American Hospitals in the Twentieth Century* (New York: Basic Books, 1989), an excellent book that picks up where Rosenberg left off; and Morris J. Vogel, *The Invention of the Modern Hospital: Boston, 1870–1930* (Chicago: University of Chicago Press, 1980), an important study that outlines the development of the modern hospital by focusing on the multitude of Boston hospitals.

Histories of specific types of hospitals include: Harry F. Dowling, *City Hospitals: The Undercare of the Underpriviledged* (Cambridge: Harvard University Press, 1982), a history of hospitals owned by cities, counties, regional authorities, or less frequently states, from the founding of the almshouse hospital in Philadelphia in 1731 to the mid-1970s; Vanessa Northington Gamble, *The Black Community Hospital: A Historical Perspective* (New York: Garland, 1987); Janet Golden, ed., *Infant Asylums and Children's Hospitals: Medical Dilemmas and Developments, 1850–1920* (New York: Garland, 1987); Diana Elizabeth Long and Janet Golden, eds., *The American General Hospital: Communities and Social Contexts* (Ithaca: Cornell University Press, 1989); and Kenneth M. Ludmerer, "The Rise of the Teaching Hospital in America," *Journal of the History of Medicine and Allied Sciences* 38, no. 4 (1983): 389–414.

Many histories of specific hospitals exist, some scholarly and some not. The American Hospital Association's Resource Center publishes a list of hospital histories in its collection. The list is available free of charge by writing to the American Hospital Association, Center for Hospital and Healthcare Administration History, 840 North Lake Shore Drive, Chicago, IL, 60611.

CHAPTER 3

Health Agencies and Foundations

PETER B. HIRTLE

Of the various types of nonprofit corporate bodies composing the U.S. health care system, two have historically performed the same broad range of functions: governmental health care agencies and private foundations. Both have played and, in the case of government agencies, continue to play significant roles in patient care, health care promotion, biomedical research, the education of health care professionals, and policy formulation. (Governmental agencies are also involved with the regulation of the health care system.) In addition to engaging in these functions directly, health care agencies and foundations also provide financial support for other corporate institutions (such as hospitals, universities, and research institutions) and individuals who carry out these functions. In their roles as a funding source for patient care or, in the case of health care agencies, as a provider of patient care, agencies and foundations are an important component of the U.S. health care system.[1] Their contributions to that system are considered in this chapter in two major sections: federal, state, and local agencies with their broader responsibilities are addressed first, followed by an analysis of foundations.[2]

GOVERNMENTAL AGENCIES

The United States, unlike most other industrial nations, lacks a centralized national health system. The absence of such a system in the United States, however, does not mean that health care is unimportant to the government. Federal agencies are active in every function of the U.S. health care system (see Table 3–1). Furthermore, the level of government involve-

TABLE 3–1 Representative governmental health agencies in the U.S. health care system

Functions of the U.S. Health Care System

Agency	Health Care Delivery		Biomedical Research	Education	Regulation/Policy Formulation	Provision of Goods/Services
	Patient Care	Health Promotion				
Federal	VA	CDC	NIH	USUHS	FDA	—
State	Spring Grove State Hospital of Maryland	Arkansas Dept. of Health, Div. of Health Education and Promotion	McArdle Laboratory for Cancer Research (Ind.)	Oregon Health Sciences University	Indiana Statewide Health Coordinating Council	—
Local	Cook County (Ill.) Hospital	Pierce County Health Council, Tacoma, Wash.	Public Health Research Institute (N.Y.)	Prince George's (Md.) Community College, Medical Record Technician Program	Baltimore Dept. of Health, Research and Planning Section	—

Abbreviations: VA, Veterans Administration; CDC, Centers for Disease Control and Prevention; NIH, National Institutes of Health; USUHS, Uniformed Services University of the Health Sciences; FDA, Food and Drug Administration.

ment with health care is significant. American governments (federal, state, and local) are the single largest source of funds spent each year on health care: in 1990 $282.6 billion, or 42.4 percent of the total expenditure on health in the United States, came from public funds.[3] Federal and local governments were the most important source of funding for health services and supplies expenditures, which include outlays for goods and services relating directly to patient care and public health plus expenses for administering the programs, providing 33.1 percent of such funding.[4]

In addition to funding certain activities of other entities, governmental agencies in the United States employ over 1.6 million people in direct patient care.[5] They also regulate private providers and health-related industries, and recently they have taken an increased role in establishing standards for care and judging compliance with them, and in planning for the general delivery of health services. Some governmental agencies are active in health promotion, while others support biomedical research and education. Despite the lack of a centralized national health care system, governmental health care agencies play an important role in defining the nature and activities of the health care system in the United States.

FUNCTIONAL ANALYSIS

Governmental agencies address almost all the functions of the U.S. health care system. The only exception is that they do not generally provide goods and services (other than insurance services). In the rare instances in which governmental agencies do provide products to the health care system, it is usually because the commercial market for the products is so small that the private sector cannot effectively address the need. Of the remaining functions of the health care system in which governmental health care agencies are actively involved, the importance of their role varies. Health care agencies play a dominant role in regulation and policy formulation, in health promotion, and biomedical research. Their activities in support of patient care and the education of health care professionals, while significant, complement similar activities in the private sector.

Almost as important as the direct involvement of governmental agencies with the functions of the U.S. health care system is their role in financing activity carried out by other groups. The amount of money spent by the federal government on direct patient care in federal facilities, for example, is dwarfed by the amount paid by the government through the Medicare program to other health care providers. Similarly, much more is spent on funding research outside of the federal government (extramural programs) than on the federal government's internal (intramural) research programs. Although funding by governmental agencies of health care activities does not constitute a separate function in the analysis followed in this book, funding does have serious implications for the kinds of record generated by those agencies, and will be considered in this chapter where appropriate.

The involvement of governmental agencies with health care takes place on three levels: federal, state, and local. The functions of health care agencies at each level are not distinct; governmental health care agencies at each of the three levels may provide patient care, fund or conduct biomedical research, promote health, formulate policy, regulate health care, or educate health care professionals. As a consequence, governmental agencies occasionally duplicate each other's efforts, while other activities may fall between the cracks and be left unaddressed. Furthermore, identical functions are often performed by different agencies in different states or even within a state.[6]

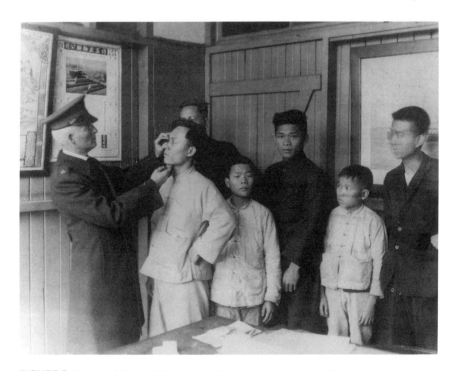

FIGURE 3–1 A Public Health Service physician inspecting Chinese immigrants in 1924. Medical inspection of aliens was one of the important early activities of this federal health agency. *Source:* National Library of Medicine, Bethesda, Md.

To understand how a system so irrational in structure and inefficient in its use of resources developed, we must understand the factors that brought it into existence. The nature of governmental involvement with health care is shaped by a combination of legal and historical factors. Because the U.S. Constitution does not clearly mandate responsibility for health care, all health care activities performed by the federal government must be performed under the general stipulation that instructs the federal government to provide for the general welfare and to regulate interstate commerce. The Constitution establishes for the nation a tripartite federal government, with responsibility for health care divided among the executive, legislative, and judicial branches. Although the laws and appropriations passed by the U.S. Congress, and the judiciary's interpretation of those laws, are important to the health care system, the agencies that are usually charged with implementing the laws are located in the executive branch.

Since powers not vested in the federal government are specifically reserved to the states, state governments have played an important role in the U.S. health care system. Many states have further delegated responsibilities to local governments, establishing the third layer of government involvement with health care. Historically, state and local governments have limited their health responsibilities to protecting citizens against the dangers of community life through public sanitation and communicable disease control. Individuals, unless they are indigent, are responsible for their own health. In the absence of total governmental responsibility for health care, and in the spirit of America's belief in voluntary and private activities in support of the government, many activities that in other countries might be assumed by the government have in the United States been undertaken by voluntary organizations or private foundations.

The U.S. health care system, therefore, has developed in a decentralized, haphazard fashion. But while federal, state, and local governments may not have assumed absolute responsibility for different functions within the system, the general focus of health care agencies at the federal, state, and local levels does differ.

FUNCTIONS OF FEDERAL HEALTH CARE AGENCIES

Several key activities dominate federal involvement in the U.S. health care system. The federal government provides patient care for selected populations, formulates much of the U.S. health care policy through regulation or reimbursement criteria, engages in biomedical research and health promotion, and is a major educator. Underlying each of these functions is the federal government's role as the source of much of the U.S. health care system's basic financial support.

PATIENT CARE

Providing patient care is one of the oldest of the federal government's health care functions and at the same time one of the least established; there is still little consensus on the extent to which the federal government should care for patients. The first federal action on health care outside of the army and navy was the establishment in 1798 of the Marine Hospital Service, now known as the Public Health Service. For most of its first century of existence, the mandate of the new organization was constrained, limited only to providing medical services to merchant seaman and funded through a mandatory employment tax on their wages.[7] Providing health care to individuals was generally considered to be a state or local responsibility; seamen were deemed a federal responsibility because they were transients who could make no fair claim to the generosity of the local community.

During the past century the federal government gradually accepted the responsibility to provide patient care to other specific groups, such as native Americans, veterans, and federal prisoners, even as the Public Health Service's original function of caring for seamen was abolished. The general delivery of patient care to the population as a whole, however, remains outside the scope of the federal government's sphere of activity.

The Department of Health and Human Services (DHHS) is the federal agency most actively involved in the health care system in general and patient care in particular. As befits a department in a government that historically has not had a clear mandate to deliver health care to its people, the agency is relatively new. It is rooted in the Federal Security Agency, which was created in 1939 to bring together into one agency all of the federal programs in the fields of health, education, and social security. The Federal Security Agency was raised to cabinet-level rank and renamed the Department of Health, Education, and Welfare in 1953; with the creation of a separate Department of Education in 1979, the DHHS was established.[8]

The DHHS is divided into four major operating divisions: the Social Security Administration, the Health Care Financing Administration, the Administration for Children and Families, and the Public Health Service. As the principlal sources for funding, the Social Security Administration and the Health Care Financing Administration have an indirect impact on the U.S. health care system. The Public Health Service and its component agencies have the greatest direct impact on health care.

The Health Resources and Services Administration (HRSA), one of the component agencies of the Public Health Service, is the primary focus for patient care programs within the federal government. In addition to providing support for efforts to improve the education of health professionals, HRSA provides services to specific groups through demonstration grants and direct patient care programs. Among the activities supported by HRSA are the Community Health Centers program, the Bureau of Prisons medical programs, and the Gillis W. Long Hansen's Disease Center in Carville, Louisiana. The Indian Health Service, formerly a part of HRSA, is now an independent agency within the Public Health Service. Its function is to provide patient care to native American and Alaskan natives through a network of hospitals, health centers, and clinics. The Substance Abuse and Mental Health Services Administration, another agency within the Public Health Service, supports demonstration programs in the treatment of substance abusors and people with mental or emotional difficulties.

Patient care is provided by agencies outside the DHHS as well. The Department of Defense is an important provider of patient care, operating an extensive system of medical facilities that provide treatment to active duty and retired military officers. In addition, the military funds the Civilian Health and Medical Program of the Uniformed Services, the system that supports patient care for entitled beneficiaries in nonmilitary hospitals. The Veterans Administration, an independent cabinet-level agency, operates the largest centrally run hospital system in the United States. It is intended to meet the medical needs of veterans who have service-related disabilities, are aged 65 and over, or are medically indigent.

Despite a historical reluctance on the part of federal governmental agencies to be involved in direct patient care and the limits on eligibility for treatment in federal facilities, delivery of medical services to individuals has become an important federal activity.

HEALTH PROMOTION

In contrast to patient care, the general promotion of public health has long been viewed as a federal function. Beginning with quarantine restrictions in the nineteenth century, the federal government has developed a number of ways to foster the general public health while leaving most patient care activities to the states or to individuals themselves. Health promotion activities occur in many federal agencies and take a variety of forms.

The Centers for Disease Control and Prevention (CDC), headquartered in Atlanta, Georgia, is the national agency primarily responsible for disease prevention, with a focus on infectious disease. The CDC directs quarantine programs, investigates outbreaks of previously unrecorded diseases, develops health education programs, sets standards for clinical laboratories, provides grants to states for local preventive campaigns, and conducts active research programs at home and abroad. CDC scientists, for example, were the first to identify Legionnaires' disease. The CDC led the campaign to eliminate smallpox from the world, and the first published notice of infection with the human immunodeficiency virus (HIV), the retrovirus associated with autoimmune deficiency syndrome, appeared in a CDC epidemiological report.

Outside of the DHHS, the U.S. Department of Agriculture (USDA) is involved with human as well as animal and plant health. Nutrition in particular has been a concern of the USDA, which administers the Women and Infant Care and Food Stamp programs. Both programs were established to combat the harmful effects of malnutrition. In addition, in the interest of public health, the USDA inspects meat and dairy products and promotes proper nutrition. The Department of Labor administers the Occupational Safety and Health Administration (OSHA), which seeks to develop and enforce workplace safety and health standards.

BIOMEDICAL RESEARCH

Perhaps in no area has federal involvement with health care been as productive as in the area of biomedical research. Federal scientists identified the causes and treatment of diseases such as pellagra, hookworm, tularemia, and Legionnaires' disease; dentists working in the Public Health Service were among the first to note the beneficial effects of fluoride on teeth and to push for the general fluoridation of water; and federal scientists led in developing an understanding of and treatment for HIV infection. Furthermore, as was noted earlier, the federal government is a major source of the funding for research carried on by others in universities, hospitals, and research institutes.

The most important agency in the federal government devoted to biomedical research is the National Institutes of Health (NIH). The primary function of the NIH is basic biomedical research, which is conducted in seventeen research institutes, one hospital, and numerous supporting centers and divisions.[9] Through its extensive extramural grant program, the NIH supports most fundamental clinical research in this country and, through its visiting scientist programs, serves as an important center for diffusing biomedical knowledge worldwide. The intramural and extramural research programs of the NIH together account for almost two thirds of all federal investment in biomedical research.

Biomedical research is also carried on in a number of different agencies both within and outside of the DHHS. Within the DHHS, the CDC maintains a large intramural research structure dedicated to investigating the source of disease outbreaks, and the newest Public Health Service agency, the Agency for Health Care Policy and Research, funds projects to ensure the most cost-effective use of health resources. Outside the DHHS, the Department of Defense maintains several important research institutes focusing on medical fields of particular concern to the military, such as tropical and arctic medicine. The Environmental Protection Agency (EPA) conducts research on the harmful effects of air, water, and ground pollution and seeks to implement the results of its studies through legislation and regulation. The Department of Energy has established laboratories investigating the effect of radiation on humans and, in support of its research efforts, is playing a key role in the current project to map the human genome. GENBANK, for example, one of the first molecular sequence data banks, began at a national laboratory run by the Department of Energy in New Mexico.[10]

POLICY FORMULATION AND REGULATION

Almost every federal agency concerned with health care is also involved in regulation and policy formulation. In some agencies, regulation is the primary function. Most notable in this regard is the Food and Drug Administration (FDA), one of the agencies that compose the Public Health Service. The FDA is charged with protecting the public from the dangers of poorly manufactured or ineffective pharmaceuticals, medical devices, radiological equipment, foods, and food additives. The FDA evaluates new products before they are marketed to ensure their safety and efficacy; periodic inspection after marketing helps ensure the continued safety of the products. To support its work, the FDA maintains an extensive set of laboratories and a criminal investigations unit, but it also relies heavily on the self-reporting of the companies involved.

The FDA's stringent regulatory requirements are frequently a source of controversy, as is the alleged failure of the agency to enforce them. A decision about the safety of silicon breast implants, a food additive such as saccharin, or grapes from Chile can keep the agency in the news for weeks. Because both personal and financial risks are involved with every decision, the volume of records generated by these FDA decisions is substantial. A single new drug application submitted by a pharmaceutical company seeking FDA approval may contain from 10,000 to over one million pages.[11] Because of the size of the applications, the FDA has been one of the federal agencies pioneering the use of digital optical storage media for the management of records.

A second, less overt form of regulation and policy formulation has emerged as a product of the federal government's role as the primary source of reimbursement for patient care expenditures, especially through the Medicare and Medicaid programs. Medicare is a nationwide health insurance program designed to help pay for hospital costs, nursing home care, physician services, and prescription drugs for the elderly, individuals receiving social security disability payments, and people with end-stage renal disease. Medicaid is a federally aided, state-operated program that provides medical benefits for certain low-income people of all ages in need of medical care. Both programs were enacted in 1965, by Titles 18 and 19 of the Social Security Act. These two programs now account for most federal health care expenditures—$175.9 billion in 1990.[12]

Both Medicare and Medicaid are modeled on private insurance programs; benefits and services are bought from private vendors, with the government itself providing few benefits. Medicare and Medicaid are primarily transfer programs. The regulations they issue are necessary for them to carry out their primary mission—supervising the administration of private or state-run health programs that are funded in part with federal dollars. As a purchaser of patient care, the government sets standards that providers must meet before public funds will be paid to them.[13] Hence the state-run programs must set payment guidelines and standards of performance for hospitals and other patient care providers, establishing to a large degree the nature and extent of medical care given in this country—in other words, formulating health care policy. For example, beginning in 1972 the federal government authorized and financed 182 professional standards review organizations (PSROs). Before federal funds could be received for hospital services, the PSROs had to review hospital records to see if hospitals were providing more care than was necessary. The PSROs were later revised into a smaller number of professional review organizations (PROs) and given the task of reviewing hospital services with the emphasis on minimizing inaccurate diagnostic data and unnecessary admissions.[14] "The requirements for review of hospital stays by PSROs and PROs," as one analyst has recently noted, "have subjected physicians to far more scrutiny of their practice than was previously the case. These requirements . . . have obliged physicians and hospital personnel to be more diligent and detailed in making entries in medical records and to document the reasons for medical decisions more extensively than before."[15] The result in hospitals and physicians' offices has been a massive increase in the volume of official patient records.[16] Much of the structure of the modern hospital, the activities which it performs, and the documentation generated in the performance of these activities have been shaped by the payment policies issued by the Health Care Financing Administration (the agency that administers most federal programs for the reimbursement of patient care). Usually, if Medicare or Medicaid refuses to pay for a certain procedure, an extended hospital stay, or an experimental drug, these options are not offered to the patient. As containment of spiraling health care costs becomes an ever-greater priority, it is likely that the Health Care Financing Administration will play a greater role in indirectly regulating the U.S. health care system.

EDUCATION

Although most education of health care personnel in the United States takes place in nonfederal institutions, federal agencies do play a small but important role. The government maintains its own medical school, the Uniformed Services University of the Health Sciences. At the NIH, CDC, EPA, and other research institutions, the government manages a series of pre- and postdoctoral and other postprofessional research and training programs. These institutions also develop many specialized educational tools as part of the continuing education of health service professionals. The federal government has also funded students during times of perceived shortages of health professionals. During World War II the Cadet Nurse Corps was established within the Public Health Service to pay for the education of nurses in approved schools of nursing; over 169,000 students were admitted to the program during its five-year existence.[17] In the 1960s and 1970s fear of an anticipated shortage of physicians led to a direct capitation program whereby medical schools were given subsidies in proportion to the number of students enrolled in their programs.[18] Although governmental support of general medical education in universities has decreased greatly, the government remains an important source of financial support for medical education at institutions outside of the federal structure.

PROVISION OF GOODS AND SERVICES

Given the size of federal expenditures for health care, it is not surprising that the federal government is directly or indirectly the single largest purchaser of health care goods and services. The federal government is not itself, however, a major provider of goods and services. One exception is a program to provide rare or experimental drugs. In 1981, for example, pentamidine was distributed only by the federal government. An upsurge in requests for it was one of the first signs alerting the government to the presence of a deadly new disease, later identified as HIV infection.[19]

THE RECORDS OF FEDERAL AGENCIES IN THE NATIONAL ARCHIVES AND RECORDS ADMINISTRATION

Federal agencies produce a large volume of records as they devise and implement their programs. The policy for creating, maintaining, and disposing of federal executive branch agency records is controlled by the Federal Records Act. The act recognized that most federal records—95 percent or more, according to the National Archives and Records Administration—are of little potential historical value. A small percentage, however, are likely to be of enduring importance because of their primary or secondary value, in particular their ability to adequately and properly document "the organization, functions, policies, decisions, procedures, and essential transactions of the agency."[20]

Records judged to be of enduring value are deposited in the National Archives, either in Washington, D.C., or at one of the eleven field branches. The records of health care agencies are well represented among the holdings of the archives. Separate record groups (the fundamental unit of archival organization) have been established for the DHHS (RG 468), for its predecessor agency, the Department of Health, Education, and Welfare (RG 235), and for many of its subsidiary agencies such as the Health Resources and Services Administration (RG 512), the CDC (RG 442), the Public Health Service (RG 90), the NIH (RG 443), the FDA (RG 88), the Agency for Health Care Policy and Research (RG 510), and St. Elizabeths Hospital (RG 418). The Office of the Army's Surgeon General (RG 112) and the Navy's Bureau of Medicine and Surgery (RG 52) also have their own record groups, as does the Veterans Administration (RG 15). The National Archives and Records Administration remains the single best source for historical information about the U.S. health care system.

STATE HEALTH AGENCIES

State health agencies are involved in almost all of the U.S. health care system's functions; as is the case with the federal agencies, only the provision of goods and services is an insignificant state function. Although the activities of the state health agencies may be in the same functional areas as the federal government, their emphasis is different. Historically, the responsibility for the general health, safety, and welfare of the population rested with the states, not with the federal government. Whereas the federal government does not provide patient care to the general population, state health agencies have themselves either developed programs in this area or delegated responsibility for such programs to local governments. In addition, state health agencies have placed a greater emphasis on health promotion activities. Much medical education is based in state universities, and the states have played an ever-increasing role in regulation. Biomedical research, a major function of the federal government, is of secondary importance at the state level except for research at state-sponsored universities.

Although these broad generalizations about the functions performed by state health agencies hold true for almost all states, how these functions are carried out, the specific agency that is assigned the function, and the relative importance of the functions vary from state to state. Each state has developed a unique health care system structure reflecting its particular history, economic conditions, and health problems. Thus, fifty-five organizational schemes for state health functions have evolved (one for each state, the District of Columbia, and the territories of American Samoa, Guam, Puerto Rico, and the Virgin Islands).[21]

Despite such diversity, some generalizations about the common functions of state health care agencies can be made. The Association of State and Territorial Health Officers (ASTHO) defines a generic "State Health Agency" as "the Agency vested with primary responsibility for public health within their jurisdictions." This generally means that the state health agency is responsible for "setting statewide public health priorities, carrying out national and state mandates, responding to public health hazards, and assuring access to health services for under-served state residents."[22] In Maryland, for example, the state agency is the Department of Health and Mental Hygiene. ASTHO surveys have further defined six core programmatic activities found in almost every state health agency: personal health, environmental health, health resources, laboratory services, general administration and services, and funding for local health department activities outside the programmatic areas listed. Services in these programmatic areas may be delivered through the state agency itself, local health departments, or a combination of the two.

PATIENT CARE

Almost all state health agencies provide patient care, which constitutes the bulk of their expenditures. Of the $9.5 billion spent by state health agencies in fiscal year 1989 for direct health care expenditures and in grants to local officials, three fourths went for personal health activities.[23] Most states support two types of programs: ambulatory care for public health concerns and institutional care for certain long-term conditions.

Ambulatory services are often conducted in conjunction with local health departments, and the programs frequently target individuals with low incomes. Maternal and child health care, including prenatal and postnatal care, family planning, and immunization, are common activities. Dental health programs, especially preventive measures such as fluoridation of water supplies, and communicable disease control programs, including immunization and the control of sexually transmitted and other infectious diseases, are also features of most state health agencies.

Institutional services are directed at long-term, chronic conditions, the treatment of which is beyond the financial capabilities of private insurance or individuals. Tuberculosis hospitals, now rare, were a prevalent example of state-sponsored institutional support of individuals with chronic disease.[24] Sixteen state health agencies operate public hospitals, long-term care facilities, or other types of in-patient care facilities.[25] Other states sponsor care for the handicapped, including programs for handicapped children, people with speech, physical, or occupational disabilities, and individuals who can be treated at home.

As with the federal government, the reimbursement for patient care delivered by private hospitals and physicians is also an important activity of state health agencies, accounting for the lion's share of the state health budget. Foremost among the reimbursement programs is Medicaid. Although the federal government defines the range of coverage available under Medicaid and provides significant funding, Medicaid is administered at the state level. States may decide whether or not to participate in Medicaid (all currently do) and choose which specific programs they will offer beyond the basic health insurance for individuals receiving public assistance.[26] States vary widely in what they will cover under Medicaid, and any coverage beyond the scope of the federal program becomes the responsibility of the state. In sum, states have tremendous discretion in designing their Medicaid programs.

HEALTH PROMOTION

State involvement in pubic health began with attempts to control communicable diseases and to ensure a safe food and water supply through sanitation. Such activities remain at the heart of most state health agencies' activities. Among the activities performed by the states in this area are the following: consumer protection and sanitation, especially in regard to food, milk, sanitation, and zoonotic disease control (rabies, Lyme disease, etc.); water quality control, including the provision or testing of water, sewage disposal, and pollution controls; solid and toxic waste control and disposal; radiation control; air quality control; and occupational safety and health. For example, the Department of Health in Missouri's Public Health Laboratory performs a number of tests on public and private water supplies: the Chemistry Unit determines the presence of minerals, nitrates, pesticides, and other chemicals in the water, and the Environmental Bacteriological Unit tests for the presence of coliform bacteria.

POLICY FORMULATION AND REGULATION

One of the first activities undertaken by states to understand the nature of disease in their communities and to promote better health was collecting and disseminating health and vital statistics. In recent years the role of state health agencies in analyzing and controlling state health resources has increased dramatically. The National Health Planning and Resources Development Act of 1974 requires that each state designate one agency as the state health planning and development agency; in most cases this is the state health agency. In addition many states have a state health coordinating council.

State health agencies may assist with the construction of new health facilities, coordinate the development of emergency services, and provide clinical laboratory services. In particular, they may require that a "certificate of need" be acquired before any new hospital construction takes place or expensive new equipment is purchased. The certificate attests to the fact that more hospital capacity or technology (a magnetic resonance imaging machine, for example) is needed. State health agencies may also regulate pharmacies, clinical laboratories, blood banks, and ambulance service. In addition, states license and regulate health professionals and support personnel, directly influencing the type and level of service available in each state. All states, for example, set certain minimum standards of training, and many require participation in a continuing education program as a prerequisite for continued licensure. Finally, most states regulate the private health insurance industry, and some regulate health maintenance organizations. Some mandate that certain minimum benefits be included in each insurance plan, and many have insurance commissioners who oversee the activity of insurance companies in the state.

EDUCATION

Many states have established or fund schools for the training physicians, nurses, dentists, and veterinarians as part of the state higher education system, and all states have courses at some level in the educational system (including community colleges) for training health personnel. Over half of the medical schools in the United States, for example, are part of a state university system; in addition, many private schools,or students attending them, receive some state support. In some states, students receive financial aid for their professional education in exchange for a commitment to practice for a specified period in underserved communities.

BIOMEDICAL RESEARCH

In 1989 state and local governments spent over $1.3 billion on health research and development.[27] Most of the money came from the states, and much of it was directed to state universities. All state medical schools have active programs for biomedical research, although the nature, direction, and search for funding of individual projects is normally left to the discretion of the individual investigator. The association of biomedical research with commercial and technological advancement has led many states to develop biotechnology and other centers for applied biomedicine. Although to date state support has primarily been of research infrastructure, in the future states may play a more direct role in supporting biomedical research.[28]

THE RECORDS OF STATE AGENCIES IN STATE ARCHIVES

State archival agencies predate the formation of the National Archives. The Alabama Department of Archives and History, the first agency in any state specifically designated to serve as the official custodian of the state's records, was established in 1901; the National Archives did not come into existence until the National Archives Act of 1934. Subsequent development of state archives was slow; it was not until the mid-1970s that every state in the union had established a formal archival program.[29]

Despite the comparatively long existence of some state archives, the management of state governmental records is often deficient. As the Report of the Committee on the Records of Government noted:

> [M]any state archivists have only a general estimate of the number of state government records outside of the archival system. In some states, less than a third of the agencies have been touched by current records management procedures. Other state archivists acknowledge that weak

agency liaison is the rule rather than the exception in their programs. In many instances, state agencies simply keep their own records. In Pennsylvania, for example, the records center reported that of the four thousand series of records scheduled for transmittal, only twelve hundred were actually in the records center. Discussing this issue with the Committee, one state archivist stated unequivocally that most state records either are not preserved or are preserved by accident.[30]

If the records of a state government agency run the risk of being lost, as recent surveys have suggested, records from health care agencies are particularly at risk. As noted earlier, much of the work of health care agencies in the states involves the direct provision of health care service. Records from these agencies frequently include information of a private nature concerning patients at mental hospitals, state-run clinics, and other state-sponsored agencies. Access to the records must be carefully controlled and limited, further limiting their potential use in an archival repository. In Michigan, for example, the Department of Mental Health was unwilling, for legal and ethical reasons, to transfer the patient records of the Ionia State Hospital for the Criminally Insane to the state archives when the hospital closed. After diligent negotiation with the department on the mechanisms by which access would be provided to the material, the state archives was able to reach an agreement with the department. Since then the records of nine other state mental hospitals have also been accessioned. The efforts of the Michigan state archives in this instance, however, appear to be unique; one must conclude that in many other states similar records would either remain with the parent agency or be destroyed.[31] Recent work on access to medical records indicates that the problems associated with the confidential nature of state medical records can be overcome, suggesting that this may in the future be less of an impediment to the preservation of state records.[32] It should be noted that there is no need to save all the patient records of every mental hospital in the United States. What the Michigan example illustrates, however, is some of the impediments to efficient retention of state health agency records.

LOCAL HEALTH AGENCIES

Defining exactly what a local health department is and how many there are in the United States is no easy task. C. A. Miller, using the definition of a local health department as "an administrative and service unit of local or state government, concerned with health, employing at least one full-time person and carrying some responsibility for the health of a jurisdiction smaller than a state," concluded in 1977 that there were between 1,073 and 2,073 local health agencies in the country.[33] ASTHO, using a similar definition, concluded in 1981 that there were 3,264 local health departments in forty-four states and territories, and no substate units in twelve other states and territories. More recently, the Public Health Foundation has concluded that there are nearly 3,000 official local health departments providing direct community health services.[34]

Because of the disparity in definitions and numbers, it is difficult to describe accurately the universe of local health departments. Nevertheless, certain generalizations can be made. Local health activities center on health promotion, broadly defined. Haven Emerson in 1945 identified the six basic activities of local public health work, and all fall within our definition of health promotion: vital statistics collection, communicable disease control, environmental sanitation, support of public health laboratories, maternal and child health promotion, and health education.[35] In practice, the local health agency is often responsible for childhood immunizations, restaurant inspections, urban rat control, and rabies control. In addition, local health departments are usually responsible for providing patient care to the poor, either in community health centers, clinics, or general hospitals. For example, the clinics of the Madison, Wisconsin, Department of Public Health offer to residents of the city services such as health advice, immunizations, dental care, and testing for sexually transmitted diseases. Of particular importance are the services they provide to immigrants and participants in the Women, Infants, and Children Program. Community-sponsored hospitals can range in size from a few beds to hundreds of beds. The 926-bed Cook County (Illinois) Hospital is an example of a large community hospital. The activities of local health agencies may be carried out independently or performed in partnership with or as a subagency of the state health department.

Local health agencies are minimally involved with functions of the U.S. health care system other than health promotion and patient care. At one time municipal laboratories were important sources of biomedical research. The most notable example is the former city laboratory that has become the New York Public Health Research Institute in New York City. Under the directorship of Hermann Biggs and W. H. Park, the laboratory was an important center for bacteriological investigation. Today the many universities in New York City have assumed the local biomedical research function. The patient care function involves some local health agencies in medical education, as many general hospitals are affiliated teaching hospitals of medical schools. And local governments are able to regulate certain medical services through zoning laws, business regulations, and the establishment of local health and safety codes. Health promotion and patient care remain, however, the major functions common to most local health agencies.

RECORDS OF LOCAL HEALTH AGENCIES

Although no formal assessment of the extent of documentation available in municipal and local archives has ever been conducted, it is likely that even fewer records relating to local health agencies have been preserved at the local level than at the state level. In his manual for local records officers, H. G. Jones noted that "a great majority of the political subdivisions in the United States—counties, towns, cities, special-purpose districts, etc.—remain without a[n archival] program of their own and receive little effective assistance from professionals at a higher level of government."[36] The situation for health records within the few jurisdictions that do maintain archives may even be worse, given the traditional lack of interest in health records. Jones provided a brief subject analysis of local records "most commonly of interest to researchers."[37] Health records are not found among them.

Local authorities have traditionally drawn on three possible avenues for preserving their records: establishing a local archives, transferring material to other repositories, such as historical societies, and transferring material to state agencies. In his book on local records, Bruce Dearstyne recommends that each jurisdiction establish its own municipal or local archives.[38] A government-maintained local archives is the most likely to have complete holdings of local records, and preserving records in their context is an important component of local practice. Both Baltimore and Philadelphia, for example, have established archives rich in local health records, reflecting the importance of American medical practice in both cities. The records for Baltimore's Health Department date from 1798, just five years after governmental involvement with health in the city began. Initial governmental interest was in quarantine and infectious disease control, but over time municipal involvement with health expanded. During the twentieth century, the agency became responsible for inspecting food, monitoring occupational safety, enforcing housing hygiene and regulating environmental quality. Starting in the 1960s, the department began supervising programs relating to child health, clinics, mental health, and addictions. Philadelphia's archives contains minutes and other records of its Board of Health and the Department of Public Health. The records of many of the clinics and hospitals managed by the city, including the Philadelphia General Hospital and the Philadelphia Nursing Home, are also retained.[39]

Yet, while the existence of a locality-sponsored archives may, as Dearstyne recommends, be the best way to protect the completeness and context of the records, the experience in Baltimore and Philadelphia suggests that even the presence of a municipal archives may not be sufficient to preserve records. As of 1984, the bulk of Baltimore's records predate World War I. Twentieth-century records, the guide notes, are "varied and small in volume." In Philadelphia the situation is similar. Although records for the early period of the city's history are relatively complete, record schedules for modern records may be outdated, placing the bulk of modern city records at risk. Fortunately, Philadelphia will shortly begin a grant-funded reevaluation of city record schedules, and new schedules that better reflect the nature and importance of modern records will be established.[40]

Baltimore City has also transferred medical records to other institutions or agencies. The records of the city's infectious disease hospital, Sydenham Hospital, for example, are housed at the National Library of Medicine. Because the collection was too large to preserve in its entirety, a sample of every tenth patient register volume was made. This example illustrates the danger of transferring records to other agencies or repositories: there is no assurance that the collection will be retained as a whole. Transferring records to either a state or private repository may be acceptable if the alternative is destruction, but if possible, it should be avoided.

The examples of Baltimore and Philadelphia indicate the weaknesses of even the best local records programs. Local records are invaluable as sources for documenting public health efforts, and selected records are worthy of preservation. Jones and Dearstyne have attempted to draw the attention of local government officials to the importance of these records, and it is hoped that local records will in the future receive more of the attention they deserve.

FOUNDATIONS

A foundation is defined by the Foundation Center as a "nongovernmental, nonprofit organization with its own funds (usually from a single source, either an individual, family, or corporation) and a program managed by its own trustees and directors, which was established to maintain or aid educational, social, charitable or other activities serving the common welfare, primarily by making grants to other nonprofit organizations."[41] The first charitable foundation in the United States was established in 1867, when George Peabody established the Peabody Fund. The period since World War II has seen an explosive growth in their numbers.

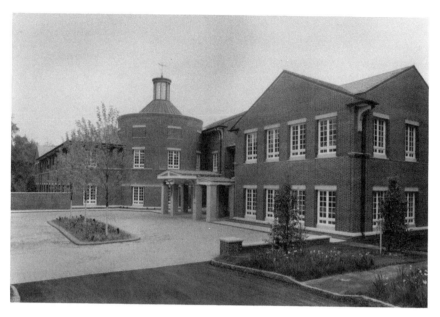

FIGURE 3–2 Headquarters of the Howard Hughes Medical Institute, the world's largest private charitable organization, in Chevy Chase, Maryland, 1993. *Source:* Howard Hughes Medical Institute; William K. Geiger, photographer

Today there are over 31,000 private foundations, ranging in size from large national foundations such as the Ford, Rockefeller, and Carnegie foundations to small local foundations. In interest and scope of activity they are similar to governmental agencies because foundations, too, act on national, state, and local levels. The Foundation Center distinguishes four common types of foundation:

- Independent foundations, usually established by an individual or family and operating with a broad charter;
- Community foundations, publicly supported organizations that derive their funds from many donors and that usually limit their giving program to their immediate area;
- Corporate foundations, established by corporations to distribute tax-free up to 10 percent of their profits; and
- Operating foundations, designed primarily to operate a specific research, social welfare, or other program.

Foundations with a special interest in health and medicine compose a large percentage; of the 31,000 foundations in the United States, more than 2,500 have a history of awarding grants relating to health matters. In 1991 almost 16 percent of all foundation grants were for health care programs or for the education of health professionals, the second largest expense category after support of schools and colleges.[42] The largest private charitable organization in the world is the Howard Hughes Medical Institute, with assets of over $6.4 billion.[43] The W. K. Kellogg Foundation, with assets of $4.2 billion, and the Robert Wood Johnson Foundation, with assets of $2.6 billion, are two other prominent foundations primarily interested in medical topics. The Rockefeller Foundation and the Commonwealth Fund, established in 1918 by the Harkness family, are two foundations that are historically important in funding aspects of the U.S. health care system.[44]

FUNCTIONS OF HEALTH-RELATED FOUNDATIONS

The primary activity of a foundation, as noted in the previous section, is to make grants to other nonprofit institutions. Foundations provide the money to maintain and support institutions active in all functions of the U.S. health care system and at one time were even active in performing those functions themselves. Many foundations, for example, were initially established to provide *patient care* to the community's indigent. This was usually accomplished by funding a local hospital or clinic, although occasionally a foundation might have employed its own physicians to provide patient care. On the national level, the Commonwealth Fund funded the construction and maintenance of hospitals in some rural areas. Through the use of demonstration projects, other foundations supported the development of local health units, resulting in a concomitant improvement in the health of the surrounding population.

Over time, however, the involvement of foundations in direct patient care has decreased. In many instances when clinics and demonstration projects begun by a foundation proved to be beneficial, governmental agencies developed the programs further. The Commonwealth Fund's support of rural hospitals, for example, served as a model for federal involvement in rural hospital construction with the Hill-Burton Act of 1946.[45] The great remaining challenge in patient care—providing patient care to the indigent or uninsured—is, however, beyond the resources of even the richest foundations. Only a few foundations still fund innovative demonstration programs in patient care, while most have shifted their emphasis to health promotion or policy analysis.

Many of the resources that foundations once committed to direct patient care have instead been spent on funding *health promotion*. Health promotion itself has always been an important function of health foundations. The eradication of hookworm in the South, for example, was primarily a result of the sanitary efforts of the Rockefeller Foundation.[46] More recently, the Robert Wood Johnson Foundation and the Kaiser Foundation have sponsored reporting on health care issues in the news media.

Foundations have historically had a major influence on *biomedical research*. Early in this century, before the funding of biomedical research was an accepted governmental function, foundations played an important role in the scientific advance of medicine.[47] Of course, the scale of foundation support for both is small in comparison to governmental support. In 1989, for example, the Howard Hughes Medical Institute expended $197 million for biomedical research and private foundations another $82 million, whereas the NIH spent over $6.7 billion on health research and development.[48] Nevertheless, the contribution to biomedical research of foundations like the Hughes is important. The Howard Hughes Medical Institute, for example, provided seed money to support early efforts to map portions of the human genome; only after their efforts helped build support for the project could NIH get budgetary authority for the project and establish the National Center for Human Genome Research.[49] Other foundations have given similar support to early fundamental work in the basic life sciences.

Medical education is the area where foundations have perhaps had the greatest influence. No foundation maintains its own medical school, and the funding of training for individuals is limited. But foundations have initiated a number of studies that have fundamentally changed the nature of medical education in this country. For example, the Flexner report on medical education (1910), which set out standards for modern medical education in the United States, was funded by the Carnegie Foundation; and the Rockefeller Foundation, through its General Education Board, provided the funds that enabled a number of universities to implement the recommendations embodied in the report. More recently, foundations have supported studies on reform of medical school curricula. The Alfred P. Sloan Foundation and the Josiah P. Macy Jr., Foundation in particular have worked to increase educational opportunities for minorities in health care fields.

In sum, foundations, like federal, state, and local agencies, provide funding to purchase equipment and to construct, renovate, or expand health care facilities; provide operating expenses or emergency funds; support research; and educate health personnel through scholarships, in-service education programs, on-the-job training, and exhibits. The importance of foundations and the reason why their records are of particular interest to historians is the pioneering role played by foundations in all these areas. Foundations have historically had the flexibility to respond quickly to innovative ideas through the development of pilot studies or demonstration projects. Successful approaches have then been replicated on a broad scale, usually by a governmental agency.

THE RECORDS OF FOUNDATIONS

As with any institutional archives, foundation records document the activities of the sponsoring organization. In addition, the records of health foundations contain important information about individuals and other groups and organizations. As Kenneth W. Rose noted, foundation records may contain "important and often difficult-to-find information about a variety of other institutions and organizations which too often disappear without leaving any paper trail of their own. Since applicants for financial support have to explain themselves, their backgrounds, and their needs to their founders, foundation records are rich in the details of the histories of other organizations."[50]

Unfortunately, Rose's survey of the records of all foundations suggests that foundation records may be at risk. Of the 1,000 largest foundations contacted for the survey, only 394 foundations chose to respond. Of those 394, only 43 (35 percent) had deposited their records in either an in-house or external archives. The situation is even worse for foundations that fund health care activities. Of the 140 foundations identified in the survey as having a historical interest in health care, only 21 (15 percent) have formal internal or external archives programs. Six of these 21 are found at the Rockefeller Archives Center; without the efforts of this one repository, the picture would be even more bleak.

Many of the foundations that have not established formal internal or external archives programs did report that archival records are found in the general records of the foundation. Yet the completeness of these records is in question. The Josiah Macy, Jr., Foundation, for example, one of the most important foundations in the history of health care in this country, reported having administrative and correspondence files only since 1976, although it was founded in 1930. Other foundations important to the development of health care, including the W. K. Kellogg Foundation, the Alfred P. Sloan Foundation, and the Pew Charitable Trusts, did not grant permission to have their responses to the survey published in the volume, suggesting that they are unwilling to allow researchers access to their records.

Fortunately, the work of Rose and others at the Rockefeller Archives Center is an important first step in alerting foundations to the importance of their records, and the center itself is an excellent model of a well-run foundation archives. Since the publication of the survey, other foundations interested in health care have either deposited records in external repositories or have established their own archives programs. The Albert and Mary Lasker Foundation, for example, deposited the records relating to the Lasker Award, the premier American award for medical research, in the National Library of Medicine. Perhaps more important, the People-to-People Foundation, Inc., the sponsor of Project HOPE, has established an internal archives at its headquarters in Millwood, Virginia. With the assistance of a National Historical Publications and Records Commission grant, the foundation has organized its 381 cubic feet of records and published a guide to its holdings. The guide is a model for other foundations interested in establishing archives.[51] One hopes that the Rockefeller Archives Center's example, the People-to-People Foundation's guide, and this volume, will encourage more foundations to establish active archival programs.

NOTES

1. Professional and voluntary associations also perform many of the same functions as health care agencies and foundations. Their contributions are considered in Chapter 6.
2. The term "agency" frequently has a specific meaning for federal, state, and local governments, designating a governmental unit at a distinct level in the government hierarchy. In this chapter it is used generically to refer to any governmental unit (department, agency, office, branch, division, etc.).
3. National Center for Health Statistics, *Health: United States, 1991, and Prevention Profile* (Hyattsville, Md.: National Center for Health Statistics, 1991), 274.
4. Ibid., 277.
5. Charles Brecher, "The Government's Role in Health Care," in Anthony R. Kovner and contributors, *Health Care Delivery in the United States*, 4th ed. (New York: Springer Publishing Company, 1990), 297.
6. The lack of consistency in agency functions from state to state was one of the driving forces behind the creation of the RLIN Seven States Project, which tried to provide access to archival collections according to functional criteria rather than by office of origin. On the Seven States Project and its functional organization, see David Bearman, "Archives and Manuscript Control with Bibliographic Utilities: Opportunities and Challenges," *American Archivist* 52 (Winter 1989): 26–39; Robert Sink, "Appraisal: The Process of Choice," *American Archivist* 53 (Summer 1990): 452–58; and Research Libraries Group, *Government Records in the RLIN Database: An Introduction and Guide* (Mountain View, Calif.: Research Libraries Group, 1990).
7. Robert Straus, *Medical Care for Seamen: The Origin of Public Medical Service in the United States* (New Haven: Yale University Press, 1950). Other discussions of the origins of the Marine Hospital Service and its mandate to treat sailors are

found in Bess Furman, *A Profile of the United States Public Health Service, 1798–1948* (Bethesda, Md.: National Library of Medicine, 1973) and Ralph Chester Williams, *The United States Public Health Service, 1798–1950* (Washington, D.C.: Commissioned Officers Association of the United States Public Health Service, 1951).

8. *A Common Thread of Service: An Historical Guide to HEW* (Washington, D.C.: Department of Health, Education, and Welfare, 1973).

9. The categorical institutes constituting the National Institutes of Health and located on the Bethesda campus of NIH are devoted to the following subjects: Aging; Alcohol Abuse and Alcoholism; Allergy and Infectious Diseases; Arthritis and Musculoskeletal and Skin Diseases; Cancer; Child Health and Human Development; Deafness and Other Communication Disorders; Drug Abuse; Dental Research; Diabetes and Digestive and Kidney Diseases; Eyes; General Medical Sciences; Heart, Lung and Blood; Mental Health; Neurological Disorders and Stroke; and Nursing Research. The National Institute of Environmental Health Sciences, also a component part of the NIH, is located in Research Triangle Park, North Carolina.

10. Several efforts are under way to document the human genome project, supported by funds from the National Center for Human Genome Research at NIH and the National Science Foundation. The Beckman Center for the History of Chemistry has begun one such effort, and the bioethics library at Georgetown University has begun another.

11. Mark Walter, "Pharmaceuticals: An Industry Ripe for Automation," in *The Seybold Report on Publishing Systems* 22(12) (March 8, 1993), 3–12.

12. National Center for Health Statistics, *Health: United States, 1991,* 294, 297.

13. Brecher, "Government's role," 309.

14. Professional standards review organizations and their impact on hospitals are discussed in more detail in Chapter 2.

15. Brecher, "Government's Role," 311.

16. Joel Howell, "Preserving Patient Records to Support Health Care Delivery, Teaching, and Research," in Nancy McCall and Lisa A. Mix, eds., *Designing Archival Programs to Advance Knowledge in the Health Fields* (Baltimore: Johns Hopkins University Press, 1994).

17. *The United States Cadet Nurse Corps and Other Federal Nurse Training Programs* (Washington, D.C.: Public Health Service, 1950), 78. See also Philip A. Kalisch and Beatrice J. Kalisch, *The Federal Influence and Impact on Nursing* (Hyattsville, Md.: Bureau of Health Professions, Division of Nursing, 1980) (NTIS doc. HRP-0900636).

18. Lauren LeRoy and Philip R. Lee, *Deliberations and Compromise: The Health Professions Educational Assistance Act of 1976* (Cambridge, Mass.: Ballinger, 1977).

19. Randy Shilts, *And the Band Played On: Politics, People, and the AIDS Epidemic* (New York: St. Martin's Press, 1987), 54.

20. Federal Records Act, 44 U.S. Code 3101.

21. An overview of the programmatic activities and expenditures of each state health agency is provided in the Public Health Foundation's annual survey of public health agencies.

22. Public Health Foundation, *Public Health Agencies 1991: An Inventory of Programs and Block Grant Expenditures* (Washington, D.C.: Public Health Foundation, 1991), 1.
23. Ibid., 3.
24. The increased incidence of antibiotic-resistant tuberculosis in the United States may lead to the revival of tuberculosis sanatoria.
25. In some other states, such as Georgia, hospitals are operated by separate hospital authorities outside of the supervision of the state health agency. *Public Health Agencies 1991*, 7.
26. Arizona, the last state to join the Medicaid program, signed on in 1982.
27. *NIH Data Book: Basic Data Relating to the National Institutes of Health* (Bethesda, Md.: National Institutes of Health, 1991), 2.
28. An interesting analogy from the world of physics is found in Utah, where much of the recent work on cold fusion was funded by the state government.
29. Committee on the Records of Government, *Report* (Washington, D.C.: Committee on the Records of Government, 1985), 71.
30. Ibid., 20. On the poor state in general of state archives, see also Lisa B. Weber, ed., *Documenting America : Assessing the Condition of Historical Records in the States* (Atlanta: Conference of the National Historical Publications and Records Commission Assessment and Reporting Grantees, 1984).
31. Roland M. Baumann, "The Administration of Access to Confidential Records in State Archives: Common Practices and the Need for a Model Law," *American Archivist* 49 (1986): 361–363.
32. In addition to the Baumann work cited above, see also McCall and Mix, *Designing Archival Programs.*
33. C. A. Miller et al., "A Survey of Local Public Health Departments and Their Directors," *American Journal of Public Health* 67 (October 1977): 931–99.
34. *Public Health Agencies 1991*, 1.
35. Haven Emerson, *Local Health Units for the Nation* (New York: Commonwealth Fund, 1945).
36. H. G. Jones, *Local Government Records: An Introduction to Their Management, Preservation, and Use* (Nashville, Tenn.: American Association for State and Local History, 1980), 19.
37. Ibid., 136.
38. Bruce W. Dearstyne, *The Management of Local Government Records: A Guide for Local Officials* (Nashville, Tenn.: American Association for State and Local History, 1988), 110–1.
39. William G. Le Furgy, *The Records of a City: A Guide to the Baltimore City Archives* (Baltimore, Md.: City Archives and Records Management Office, 1984), 36, and John Daly, *Descriptive Inventory of the Archives of the City and County of Philadelphia* (Philadelphia: Department of Records, 1970).
40. Ibid., 37; telephone conversation with David Weinberg, Philadelphia City Archives, 27 June, 1993.
41. *National Data Book of Foundations, 1991* (New York: Foundation Center, 1991), v. The Foundation Center, a nonprofit organization founded and supported by foundations "to provide a single authoritative source of information on

foundation giving," is the best source of information on foundations (also called philanthropic foundations, charitable trusts, trusts, charitable corporations, and sometimes funds). See the *Foundation Directory* (New York: Foundation Center, 1992), xxi–xxxii.

42. *National Guide to Funding in Health,* 2nd ed. (New York: Foundation Center, 1989), v, and Ruth Kovacs, ed., *Foundation Grants Index 1993,* 21st ed. (New York: Foundation Center, 1992), xii–xiii.

43. The Howard Hughes Medical Institute is not technically a foundation under the tax code but instead is a medical research organization. Because its activities and purpose are so similar to those of foundations, it is considered with foundations in this chapter.

44. Robert J. Glaser, "The Impact of Philanthropy on Medicine and Health," *Perspectives in Biology and Medicine* 36 (1992): 46–56. This source provides a useful historical introduction to the activities of several major foundations in support of health care.

45. A. McGhee Harvey and Susan Abrams, *For the Welfare of Mankind: The Commonwealth Fund and American Medicine* (Baltimore: Johns Hopkins University Press, 1986).

46. John Ettling, *The Germ of Laziness: Rockefeller Philanthropy and Public Health in the New South* (Cambridge: Harvard University Press, 1981).

47. Barbara G. Rosenkrantz and Peter Buck, Introduction, in *Philanthropic Foundations and Resources for Health: An Anthology of Sources* (New York: Garland Publishing, 1990): xi–xix.

48. *NIH Data Book 1991,* 2.

49. George F. Cahill, Jr., and Diane R. Hinton, "Howard Hughes Medical Institute and Its Role in Genomic Activities," *Genomics* 5 (November 1989): 952–54; and Robert Mullan Cook-Deegan, "The Human Genome Project: The Formation of Federal Policies in the United States, 1986–1990," in Kathi E. Hanna, ed., *Biomedical Politics* (Washington, D.C.: National Academy Press, 1991), 99–175.

50. Kenneth W. Rose, *The Availability of Foundation Records: A Guide for Researchers* (North Tarrytown, N.Y.: Rockefeller Archives Center, 1990), IV-2–IV-3. See also Darwin H. Stapleton and Kenneth W. Rose, eds., *Establishing Foundation Archives: A Reader and Guide to First Steps* (Washington, D.C.: Council on Foundations, 1991).

51. Chuck Hill and Anne Muchoney, eds., *A Guide to the Project HOPE Archives* (Millwood, Va.: People-to-People Foundation, 1991).

SELECT ANNOTATED BIBLIOGRAPHY

Several general guides to the U.S. health care system present good overviews of the functions, activities, and roles of federal, state, and local health agencies. Among the best are Anthony R. Kovner and contributors, *Health Care Delivery in the United States* (New York: Springer Publishing Company, 1990); Florence

A. Wilson and Duncan Neuhauser, *Health Services in the United States* (Cambridge, Mass.: Ballinger, 1985); and Milton I. Roemer, *Ambulatory Health Services in American: Past, Present, and Future* (Rockville, Md.: Aspen Systems Corporation, 1981), which also contains a good overview of patient care activities of disease-specific foundations. An excellent compilation of essays on the government's role in formulating health policy is Theodore J. Litman and Leonard S. Robins, *Health Politics and Policy* (Albany, N.Y.: Delmar Publisher, 1991).

The best history on the origins of the Public Health Service (and hence federal involvement with health care) remains that by Robert Straus, *Medical Care for Seamen: The Origin of Public Medical Service in the United States* (New Haven: Yale University Press, 1950). The most recent history is Fitzhugh Mullan, *Plagues and Politics: The Story of the United States Public Health Service* (New York: Basic Books, 1989). Recent historical studies of other federal health agencies include Victoria Harden, *Inventing the NIH: Federal Biomedical Research Policy, 1887–1937* (Baltimore: Johns Hopkins University Press, 1986); Elizabeth Etheridge, *Sentinel for Health: A History of the Centers for Disease Control* (Berkeley and Los Angeles: University of California Press, 1992); and Alice Sardell, *The U.S. Experiment in Social Medicine: The Community Health Center Program, 1965–1986* (Pittsburgh: University of Pittsburgh Press, 1988).

The classic work on local health units is Haven Emerson, *Local Health Units for the Nation: A Report* (New York: Commonwealth Fund, 1945; reprinted by Arno Press, 1977). In 1973 a team at the University of North Carolina began an important project to survey the activities and organization of local health agencies. A good example of their work is C. A. Miller et al., "A Survey of Local Public Health Departments and Their Directors," *American Journal of Public Health* 67 (1977), 931–39. An excellent model history that focuses on the activities of a local health department is John Duffy, *A History of Public Health in New York City, 1625–1866* (New York: Russell Sage Foundation, 1968-[74]).

The standard work on the structure and organization of foundations is Frank Emerson Andrews, *Philanthropic Foundations* (New York: Russell Sage Foundation, 1956). The value of the archives of philanthropic foundations, including health-related foundations, has been argued by David C. Hammack in "Private Organizations, Public Purposes: Nonprofits and Their Archives," *Journal of American History* 76 (1989): 181–91. Good histories of the health activities of important foundations include A. McGehee Harvey and Susan L. Abrams, *For the Welfare of Mankind: The Commonwealth Fund and American Medicine* (Baltimore: Johns Hopkins University Press, 1986); E. Richard Brown, *Rockefeller Medicine Men: Medicine and Capitalism in America* (Berkeley and Los Angeles: University of California Press, 1979); and John Ettling, *The Germ of Laziness: Rockefeller Philanthropy and Public Health in the New South* (Cambridge: Harvard University Press, 1981).

CHAPTER 4

Biomedical Research Facilities

PAUL G. ANDERSON

Biomedical research facilities are units of the U.S. health care system devoted primarily to scientific investigations in medicine or other modes of therapeutic treatment, or to studies of the basic composition and functions of the human body. This chapter reviews the major types of biomedical research institutions and their activities. As shown in Table 1–1, biomedical research institutions are inextricably involved with most functions of the health care system. The signature function of research may not readily be distinguished from other principal functions. Many kinds of investigative units, for example, are involved in patient care. Their programs often contribute a vital part to the education (particularly postgraduate training) of health care professionals. Indirectly their influence extends still further: biomedical research findings are an essential ingredient in health promotion and policy formulation, and they make possible the manufacture and marketing of products and services worth billions of dollars annually.

Institutions in the United States devoted to biomedical research number in the thousands and include programs in the basic sciences, such as molecular biology and biophysics, as well as in the clinical sciences, such as cardiology and surgery. Units that conduct programs dedicated to developing refinements in biomedical technology within larger institutions belong equally to this category. The concept of biomedical research also includes investigations in allied health fields, such as dental medicine, nursing, and pharmacology, and in behavioral sciences, such as psychology and sociology.[1] In this chapter, the term will be used in its broadest sense.

Specialty institutions devoted to biomedical research fields are identified by a welter of generic terms, some clearly denoting a particular function or size, others seemingly devoid of meaningful association. The jargon of the National Institutes of Health (NIH), the largest of the Public Health Service branches of the Department of Health and Human Services, for example, speaks of "BIDs"—*bureaus, institutes,* and *divisions.*[2] There are also many federal research agencies bearing the name *center.* Institutions outside the government are designated by these same terms, but many others are used as well. The nonprofit sector recognizes numerous research *academies, clinics, consortiums, departments, groups, foundations, laboratories, programs,* and *units.* The commercial sector adds *companies* and *corporations.*

Unmistakable from even a casual analysis of this segment of the U.S. health care system is the fact that independent biomedical research units are far outnumbered by comparable organizations that are subdivisions of larger bodies. Fewer than one in ten are without some form of parent body. Throughout the country, there is a proliferation of specialty units within governmental agencies, hospitals, universities, and commercial companies. This is not to say that independent biomedical research institutions are a declining phenomenon. There are today, as there have been for decades, many new and vital organizations of this description. At present, however, the trend favors the development of large, conglomerate medical enterprises.[3]

Another general characteristic of research institutions, and one that is related to the frequency of their affiliated or subordinate status, is that as a rule they are neither quite as visible nor as permanent as other kinds of organizations in the U.S. health care system. Most U.S. hospitals, for example, take as part of their mission to be known as permanent community assets and often assiduously cultivate their public image through media advertising and other, more subtle public relations campaigns. Educational institutions also desire visibility to attain objectives such as the recruitment of students and the maintenance of alumni and community support. Health industry firms routinely spend millions of dollars annually to encourage the public to trust and use their products. By contrast, a public profile is deemed unnecessary, if not undesirable, for most specialty research organizations. Such units are established when intellectual motivation and funding opportunities come together, and this generally happens with far less fanfare than is heard from institutions that directly serve the public. When all their projects conclude or funding is exhausted, most research organizations, both public and private, can relatively swiftly disburse their property assets and disband.

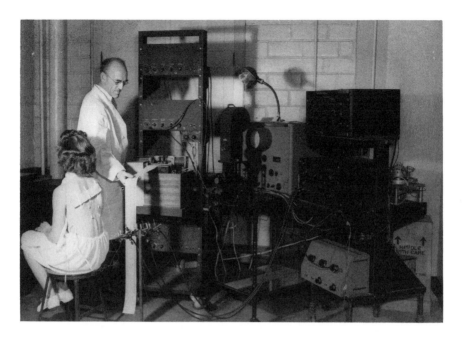

FIGURE 4–1   Dr. George H. Bishop conducts research on sensory mechanisms of skin in the Neurophysiology Laboratory, McMillan Hospital–Oscar Johnson Institute, Washington University, St. Louis, 1946. *Source:* Washington University School of Medicine Library, St. Louis

TYPES OF BIOMEDICAL RESEARCH INSTITUTIONS

The federal government has long established and operated biomedical research agencies. Every state of the union also funds agencies that conduct investigations in health-related fields. Completing the picture are varieties of investigative units that are both private and nonprofit and also many that are run for profit. Both federal and profit-making units tend to be unambiguous concerning control and funding. The investigatory branches of the Department of Health and Human Services, for example, operate totally on congressional appropriations. Their work is performed ostensibly in the public interest, and significant findings are generally divulged as soon as it is feasible. Commercial biomedical firms usually conduct research out of corporate revenues; findings from their laboratories are proprietary and disseminated according to marketing strategies.

The factors of control and funding are often more complicated in the cases of state agencies and of private, nonprofit biomedical research institutions. A large proportion of institutions in both categories depend on complicated and multilayered funding systems extending across state lines. Various federal grant programs enable state, local, and private nonprofit organizations to form special units for biomedical research. Private foundations and corporate sponsors also play a central role in sustaining nonprofit investigative organizations, both within and apart from governmental control. All of this is carried on in the public interest or, from a different perspective, in the interest of science and health.[4]

Private philanthropy accounts for what most closely approximates a legal definition of a "typical" biomedical research organization. This definition is found in a section of the Internal Revenue Code concerning the eligibility of such units to receive private donations. According to the code, an organization is a medical research organization [if it is] directly engaged in the continuous active conduct of medical research in conjunction with a hospital."[5] Under the strictest possible interpretation, the law would appear to address only those units that are subordinate sections of major health care delivery facilities. The phrase "in conjunction with a hospital," however, is generally taken to include many different levels of association with clinical institutions, among them purely intellectual and collegial connections. A broad interpretation permits wholly independent organizations engaged in health sciences research to receive donations under the code.[6] Many research units, furthermore, are eligible recipients of charitable contributions and gifts by virtue of being part of educational institutions.[7]

FEDERAL BIOMEDICAL RESEARCH LABORATORIES

The federal government operates several hundred specialized biomedical research components. These are parts of the agencies already reviewed in broader perspective in Chapter 3. The greatest number are grouped under the egis of the Public Health Service of the Department of Health and Human Services. They include the institutes and centers that compose the NIH, the divisions of the Substance Abuse and Mental Health Services Administration, and the Centers for Disease Control. They all are commonly referred to as intramural research laboratory units (i.e., operating within the "walls" of the federal government), to draw a distinction between them and the extramural research program offices operated by many of the same institutes and divisions, in which money is sent "beyond the walls." Many specialized biomedical research institutes and divisions are also to be found within the departments of Agriculture, Defense, Energy, and Veterans Affairs.[8]

Federal agencies set national standards not only because they are sources of funding, but also because they serve, at least in principle, as flagships in their respective investigative fields. At the very least, they have been centers where scientists across the country gained formative experiences and made important associations. This leadership function was particularly significant during the halcyon early years of the NIH (roughly the late 1940s through the early 1960s). In his autobiography, *For the Love of Enzymes,* the biochemist Arthur Kornberg recalls how young scientists typically exchanged positions at the NIH for appointments at other institutions, or vice versa, in the course of their careers.[9] Competition between the NIH and the world outside Bethesda for candidates to fill junior posts and postdoctoral fellowships continues to renew and strengthen these same connections. Mutual reinforcement, moreover, is perpetuated through the experiences of members of hundreds of review panels that convene at the NIH as a part of the annual grant-funding process.

Specialization renders it impossible to represent any one federal laboratory unit as typical of all that the government operates. The mammoth NIH campus in Bethesda houses the largest concentration of intramural research programs. There, to cite but one example, are located the laboratories of the Digestive Diseases Branch, Intramural Research Division, of the National Institute of Diabetes and Digestive and Kidney Diseases, one of the thirteen National Institutes of Health. This unit boasts two sections, devoted respectively to gastroenterology and to liver diseases, where scientists conduct experiments on the physiology and biochemistry of digestive disorders. A prominent example of NIH laboratories located outside Bethesda are the units administered by the Gerontology Research Center of the National Institute of Aging, in Baltimore. A wide range of investigations on the aging process and age-related disorders are conducted at the center's facilities.

Military medicine embraces numerous fields of applied biomedical research. The Letterman Army Institute of Research in San Francisco, for example, is devoted to problems related to battlefield trauma and defenses against biological and chemical weapons. The Diving Medicine Department of the Naval Medical Research Institute in Bethesda specializes in studies of decompression sickness, the use of anesthesia and other drugs below the ocean's surface, and the long-term effects of contaminants on divers. The Department of Veterans Affairs, in addition to maintaining cooperative research contracts with medical centers throughout the United States, operates its own Medical Research Service at departmental headquarters in Washington, D.C., to investigate clinical problems especially prevalent in Veterans Administration hospitals.

HOSPITAL- OR UNIVERSITY-AFFILIATED RESEARCH INSTITUTIONS

"Affiliated status" in this context covers both integral research units of hospitals and universities and research institutions that maintain cooperative arrangements with hospitals and universities. They are commonly located within both state-supported and private, nonprofit medical centers. Federal extramural funding, private philanthropy, and clinically generated revenues have contributed to make equivalent units in both ownership categories remarkably similar.

An example of an integral unit is the Bockus Research Institute in Philadelphia. Bockus is a part of the Graduate Hospital Research Center, which in turn is affiliated with the University of Pennsylvania (although not owned by the university). The institute specializes in research in cardiovascular physiology. An example of an institution with a more collateral relationship with a hospital complex is the Brain Research Center, an independent, nonprofit organization affiliated with the George Washington University School of Medicine and located at Children's National Medical Center in Washington, D.C. Research there concentrates on the role of neuropeptides in the nervous systems of children, and the center is currently running experiments in the treatment of autistic and self-injurious behavior. Not all hospital-affiliated research units, however, conduct laboratory experiments. The Sid W. Richardson Institute for Preventive Medicine of the Methodist Hospital in Houston, for example, specializes in epidemiological studies of chronic lung and heart diseases. Among its objectives are the analysis of health insurance claims and employee absentee data to evaluate preventive medicine programs.

The overwhelming majority of biomedical research institutions function within a single facility, but there are numerous exceptions. The Affiliated Children's Arthritis Centers of New England, for example, is a research organization comprised of a network of fifteen tertiary pediatric centers located throughout the region and based at the Floating Hospital of New England Medical Center in Boston. The organization conducts a series of programs on childhood rheumatic diseases, including clinical and health management research, and community education courses and workshops.

Private hospitals that house research institutes number in the hundreds. These special branches are located throughout the United States, though virtually all are found in major metropolitan areas. As noted in the previous chapter, the economic and social realities of the U.S. health care system make it difficult to operate large private hospitals outside urban centers. This is doubly true for costly research units. The investigatory divisions of the Mayo Clinic in Rochester, Minnesota, are exceptions in this regard. The Mayo Foundation continues to operate research programs in private facilities, although with extensive government support. The General Clinical Research Center at Mayo Foundation is located at St. Mary's Hospital in Rochester and is funded by the NIH's General Clinical Research Centers Program, which underwrites investigations in a wide range of clinical specialties. Other Mayo research facilities are housed at Rochester Methodist Hospital. More recently, the foundation has established group practices in Jacksonville, Florida, and Scottsdale, Arizona. A special satellite telecommunications system permits staff physicians at these locations to participate in selected research programs centered in Rochester.[10]

Academic medical centers have increasingly developed as the locations of choice for biomedical research. Minimal components for an academic medical center are a hospital and a degree training program in at least one branch of the health sciences, but this hardly suffices to describe the massive conglomerates that have emerged under this bare description in many large urban areas.[11] As with hospitals and research units, a hierarchical affiliation is not a necessity. Many institutions have been able to devise cooperative arrangements and to derive other mutual benefits from mere proximity. An outstanding example of this is the clustering of biomedical research institutions in metropolitan Houston in the vicinity of several universities and hospitals.

The biomedical research units at Boston University are typical of special investigatory divisions that have developed under the umbrellas of academic medical centers throughout the United States: the Aphasia Research Center, the Arthritis Center, the Center for Psychiatric Rehabilitation, the General Clinical Research Center, the Gerontology Center, the Health Policy Institute, the Hubert H. Humphrey Cancer Research Center, the Human Bioenergetics Laboratory, the Laboratory of Neurophysiology, the Marine Program, the Robert Dawson Evans Memorial Department of Clinical Research, and the Whitaker Cardiovascular Institute. Major university medical centers such as Boston University's are, in general, more intellectually diverse than those connected to hospitals without graduate degree programs in the health sciences. Many extend beyond biomedicine proper to allied fields in biology, bioengineering, and the social sciences. Boston University, for example, maintains a year-round research program at the facilities of the Marine Biological Laboratory in Woods Hole, Massachusetts. The fact that Boston University is privately owned has no bearing on the array of research units that it maintains or the kinds of investigations in which they engage. Numerous large state universities support comparable numbers and varieties of investigatory bodies.

INDEPENDENT NONPROFIT BIOMEDICAL RESEARCH INSTITUTIONS

A select number of private, nonprofit agencies occupy enormously influential positions at the centers of the experimental life sciences, each with numerous links to the world of clinical practice as well. Particularly illustrative of institutions in this rank are three of the oldest in the United States—the Carnegie Institute of Washington, the Cold Spring Harbor Laboratory in Cold Spring Harbor, New York, and the Marine Biological Laboratory in Woods Hole, Massachusetts.

The Carnegie Institute of Washington is a private organization with centers in several cities. In terms of biomedical research, the most notable of these centers is the Department of Embryology, founded in 1914, and located in Baltimore. The department's general research agenda is to study the "mechanism of differentiation, growth, and morphogenic processes coordinating transformation of an egg into a functional adult." The institute also operates the Carnegie Laboratories of Embryology, Davis Division, located at the University of California, Davis, specializing in investigations in embryonic development of the human brain. The division is operated under contract by the university.

The Cold Spring Harbor Laboratory, founded in 1890, is a nonprofit research organization affiliated with ten sponsoring universities but governed by its own board. It boasts a research staff numbering in the hundreds, some of whom are active in fields only tangentially related to the human health sciences. The laboratory has long been among the leading centers of work in genetics and molecular biology in the United States. Cancer investigations are another important part of its program.

Founded in 1888, the Marine Biological Laboratory is among the most venerable of the private independent research institutions. Despite the name, the laboratory is not exclusively devoted to the study of marine life but is renowned for research conducted on cell biology, neurobiology, and other areas with a human focus. The laboratory is particularly well known for its summer institute, where scientists in biomedical and related disciplines from around the world lease space to further their research projects. In addition to the arrangement with Boston University's Marine Program, the laboratory also houses a year-round research program of the University of Pennsylvania.

Some independent biomedical research institutions have small staffs and limited research budgets. Their programs may, nevertheless, be far-reaching and ambitious. The Center for Human Genetics, a nonprofit laboratory in Bar Harbor, Maine, for example, has only one permanent staff scientist. The center investigates genetic approaches to understanding and treating a variety of birth defects and congenital debilities. The Center for the Study of Anorexia and Bulimia is a nonprofit division of the Institute for Contemporary Psychotherapy in New York City and conducts studies on the prevalence, demography, etiology, and treatment of these eating disorders. Its operation is funded almost completely by clinic income. One of the best known centers for research in human sexuality is the Masters and Johnson Institute, in St. Louis. Its program includes the study of conceptive, contraceptive, and human sexual physiology, psychology, and endocrinology.

Some independent research units specialize in fields and treatments traditionally eschewed by major medical centers. The Acupuncture Research Institute, for example, is a private, nonprofit research organization in Monterey Park, California, devoted to the ancient Chinese healing art. It sponsors clinical conferences and seminars at the Queen of Angels Hollywood Presbyterian Medical Center and at Los Angeles International University. Another example is the Laban/Bartenieff Institute of Movement Studies, Inc., in New York City, which investigates applications of a form of physical therapy with roots outside any of the natural sciences. Rudolf Laban (1879–1958), an Austrian dancer and choreographer, formulated a series of principles for the understanding of body movement that were applied to therapy by a disciple, Irmgard Bartenieff (1900–1981). The institute claims that these principles have applications to psychotherapy, fitness, and sports training.

BIOMEDICAL RESEARCH AND DEVELOPMENT COMPANIES OR DIVISIONS OF COMPANIES

All profit-making enterprises in biomedical fields necessarily engage to some degree in research. Although the health industries in the United States are the subject of Chapter 7, many varieties of specialty research units within the commercial sector of the contemporary health care system will be discussed here. The similarities and close ties that exist between them and nonprofit institutions are noteworthy. Advanced work in the fields of cellular or molecular biology and genetics, for example, relies on intimate professional contacts between investigators, on one side, and suppliers of apparatus, drugs, and reagents, who are themselves scientists, on the other.[12]

Life Technologies, Inc., of Gaithersburg, Maryland, is typical of many small research and development companies that have emerged to supply NIH laboratories and extramural scientific institutions with instruments and materials relating to DNA technology and advanced clinical diagnostics. The company conducts its own research in areas such as restriction enzymes, eukaryotic transcription systems, and hepatitis B hybridization.

Synergen, Inc., of Boulder, Colorado, is an example of a firm oriented toward fields outside the health professions (e.g., applications of microorganisms in enhanced oil recovery) that has discovered applications of its research to clinical medicine (e.g., the treatment of lung disease). Some companies have been established by nonprofit institutions to exploit the commercial potential of biomedical research. A prominent example is Salk Institute Biotechnology Industrial Associates, Inc., of San Diego, which conducts research under contract with several larger firms, among them Phillips Petroleum, in selected areas of cell biology and genetics.

RESEARCH PARTNERSHIPS BETWEEN COMMERCIAL COMPANIES AND NONPROFIT INSTITUTIONS

Recent decades have witnessed extraordinary developments in partnerships between commercial companies and nonprofit institutions. A trend-setting event in this area was the $23 million contract awarded to Harvard Medical School by the Monsanto Company in 1974 to fund cancer research.[13] The essence of this and subsequent agreements, distinguishing them from totally commercial research ventures, is that industrial firms agreed to underwrite investigatory programs using the facilities and staffs of nonprofit institutions in return for a share in the rights to lucrative discoveries.[14]

Major partnerships might have developed before the 1970s had there not been a perception on the part of industry that if nonprofit organizations were recipients of federal grants or contracts and private money, all rights to discoveries would fall in the public domain. A lawsuit that has become known as the Gator-Ade case led to an important clarification of this matter. A University of Florida researcher discovered a formula for a soft drink demonstrably beneficial to athletes. After the university declined to file for a patent, the scientist contracted in 1969 with the Stokley Van Camp Company to produce the beverage. Gator-Ade proved profitable, whereupon the university belatedly filed suit to claim all royalties. The case, settled out of court, inspired the passage of Public Law 96–517 in 1980, giving nonprofit institutions and small businesses the right to retain title to inventions resulting from government grants and contracts. The legislation has opened the door to scores of joint agreements between nonprofit research organizations and small commercial biotechnology firms.

The 1980s witnessed the advent of several multi-million-dollar contracts between academic medical centers and large chemical or pharmaceutical companies which are noteworthy.[15] Massachusetts General Hospital, the largest Boston teaching hospital associated with Harvard University, was foremost among institutions of its kind to establish industrial partnerships. The German chemical firm Hoechst AG signed a contract with Massachusetts General in 1980 to create a $68 million molecular biology center. In 1989, the hospital announced an $85 million contract with Shiseido Co., Ltd., of Japan to support a center for research on skin and skin diseases. In the following year, a $36.8 million agreement was reached between the hospital and the pharmaceutical giant Bristol-Myers Squibb to establish a cardiovascular research unit.

Among universities with large research-oriented medical centers, Washington University in St. Louis set precedents for attracting huge corporate contracts. In 1981 the university agreed with Mallinckrodt, also of St. Louis, to undertake a $3.8 million research project focusing on hybridomas, artificially created cells that produce antibodies useful in the treatment of a variety of diseases. The following year, the university joined with another St. Louis chemical firm, Monsanto, to study cellular communications, particularly proteins and peptides that affect the immune system. Originally calling for $23.5 million in corporate support, subsequent renewals of the pact have augmented the total committed to nearly $100 million, earning it the distinction of being to date the most extensive research collaboration ever funded between an American company and an American university.[16]

Agreements such as these have aroused considerable controversy. Critics warned that the profit motive and the restrictions placed by the contracts on dissemination of findings and the rights to discoveries could corrupt academic medicine beyond redemption.[17] Spokespersons for the parties involved have responded by praising their agreements as model collaborative programs, contending that the rights, licenses, and royalties that academic investigators reserve for their corporate sponsors constitute a reasonable price for underwriting their work.[18] There is reason to expect that major academic-industrial partnerships will continue and expand in the future.

FUNCTIONS AND ACTIVITIES OF BIOMEDICAL RESEARCH INSTITUTIONS

Most early medical researchers in the United States were physicians who worked in relative isolation to discover new treatments or new knowledge of the human body. William Beaumont (1785–1853), to cite a well-known example of a pioneer investigator, conducted experiments on digestive physiology in his home on an isolated army post in the 1820s, focusing his attention on a single patient. To observe here that

Beaumont's world disappeared long ago is an understatement. The stark differences between biomedical research then and now underscore why today few research programs are possible without elaborate planning and support. The activities outlined here apply equally to investigations in hospitals, educational institutions, and programs of independent research institutions.

The functions and activities of biomedical research units are complicated and diverse. Nevertheless, they can be classified into a relatively few basic categories. The range of activities composing the research function is unquestionably central; patient care and education are secondary functions. Not only the core function but also certain activities composing the institutional administration function deserve archival scrutiny. Before experimentation begins, efforts must be organized to *secure funding* and *recruit personnel.* All during the operating lifetime of the unit, work is performed not only by a scientific elite but also by employees who acquire and *manage the equipment, facilities, and materials.* The *training* of junior staff members and students may be objectives requiring substantial attention and expenditures. Activities such as these represent more than a string of peripheral events, for they are the background to the research process in which investigations are proposed and justified, and results disseminated.[19]

BASIC, CLINICAL, AND APPLIED BIOMEDICAL RESEARCH

Biomedical research is typically dedicated to the pursuit of basic scientific or clinical knowledge. Rephrasing the definition with which this chapter began, the difference between basic and clinical research is the difference between studies of the functions and composition of the human body, on one hand, and investigations in medicine or other modes of therapeutic treatment, on the other. Some observers would see this difference as a health sciences version of the dichotomy common to all intellectual endeavors—distinguishing fundamental work from applied. Others discern nuances between the concepts of clinical and applied research and between therapeutic and nontherapeutic investigation. Merely having patients tested, we are reminded, is not enough to make the project practical or useful.[20]

Many distinctions between basic and clinical sciences are more theoretical than real. An ever-expanding and overlapping array of research subfields encompasses all areas of biomedical research. The basic biomedical sciences may still be known in part by academic names such as anatomy, biochemistry, genetics, microbiology, pharmacology, and physiology, all of which are subjects in the classic medical education curriculum. The identity of clinical sciences is reinforced by counterparts among common hospital services (e.g., internal medicine, surgery, anesthesiology, obstetrics/gynecology, ophthalmology, otolaryngology, neurology, psychiatry, and radiology). But beneath the intellectual matrix corresponding to the services and departments of clinical and educational institutions there is much overlap and constant change.

The 1980s and 1990s have witnessed increasing concentration on molecular and cell biological research engaged in by scientists of various departmental affiliations. Contemporary biomedicine is now conducted and expressed, as Kornberg phrased it, "in a common language of chemistry."[21] The three following examples illustrate crossovers from basic to clinical research. Certain projects to discover new treatments for epilepsy draw on the expertise of biochemists and pharmacologists in testing anticonvulsion agents; work on growth inhibitory factors by immunologists and zoologists has contributed to the effectiveness of agents inhibiting the rejection of transplanted organs; and studies of how molecules are distributed among distinctive cell regions have proved to have important applications to understanding the functions of photoreceptors in the human retina, and to yield new forms of treatment to restore impaired vision.[22]

Applied research programs in engineering and physics continually produce advances in testing and diagnostic equipment, which offer broad applications for biomedical programs. Radiology and surgery are among the fields that most frequently benefit from new technology, such as magnetic resonance imaging, positron emission tomography, and video-guided laparoscopic surgery. New synthetic materials for implants and prostheses are frequently introduced from chemical and engineering laboratories outside biomedicine. Every discipline of biomedical research has profited from technologies as various as electron microscopy, chemical microbalances and microsensors, lasers, and microchips, to name but a few. Many innovations open up new avenues for diagnostic and therapeutic investigations at the same time that they themselves are undergoing further testing and refinement.[23]

In all of biomedical research, and particularly among institutions in the nonprofit sector, collaboration regularly extends beyond institutional walls. The science writer Michael Spector described the interaction succinctly: "Researchers for the NIH, universities, and private businesses routinely join together in their attempts to develop a drug, for example, or to understand the nature of a scientific problem. Groups form and dissolve constantly, based on scientific predilection and research needs. [Leading scientists] benefit tremendously from these new protean arrangements."[24] Biomedical scientists may aspire to unique credit for major discoveries but generally acknowledge their dependence on colleagues. Meetings of professional societies, the review process for grant applications and for publication of findings, and improved technologies in medical informatics all encourage collaboration.

RESEARCH FUNCTION: FUNDING

In the 1960s and 1970s, the federal government accounted for about 60 percent of biomedical research funding, and industry accounted for 25 to 30 percent. These relative proportions of funding changed in the 1980s as industry increased its funding, especially in the areas of biotechnology and pharmaceutical research. Of the $22.6 billion spent on biomedical research in 1990, roughly 46 percent was funded by industry, 44 percent by the federal government, and 10 percent by private nonprofit foundations and other sources.[25] Industry and the federal government tend to fund different types of biomedical research. Whereas industry tends to focus on funding applied research in private laboratories, the federal government concentrates its funding on basic biomedical research projects in academic institutions and federal laboratories. As funding resources dwindle, however, governmental funding priorities may shift toward applied research.

Securing research funding requires the detailed communication of methods, objectives, and costs involved in the proposed investigations. Projects that are unsponsored—that is, projects that are supported by the internal revenues of an organization—must at very least be justified and budgeted to a degree sufficient to satisfy the scrutiny of the sponsoring medical center's overall management. Major governmental grants or contracts require lengthy applications, followed by periodic reports, audits, and other communications to funding agencies. Support from private foundations may require less paperwork than the NIH or other federal grant endowments, but they, too, entail extensive administrative preparations and oversight. Commercial ventures generally involve, in addition, extensive legal arrangements.[26]

Association with a larger organization can provide a research unit with crucial assistance in maintaining its program over time. Institutional links help to establish and promote the credentials of research programs and expedite financial operations. Universities and hospitals, for example, routinely negotiate blanket agreements with funding agencies covering all their research subsidiaries. As a result, the number of staff directly involved with grants administration and employed within the individual research units is minimized. Despite controversy over "excessive" administrative overhead charged at certain institutions (as in the widely publicized case of Stanford University), basic formulas for determining indirect costs incurred by extramural research units have been followed for decades. Many large research centers have established committees to monitor the situation and avoid possible abuses.

Competition for funding can be fierce among colleagues at competing institutions or even at the same institution. In the 1980s, the chance of being funded by the NIH decreased from 32 percent to 24 percent of submitted applications, for three reasons: (1) each grant cost more, (2) project awards covered a longer period of time, and (3) the number of high-quality applications increased.[27]

Senior scientists play a significant role in regulating the system through participation in various aspects of the peer review process. Through study sections, the formal panels summoned to advise the NIH, or through less formal advisory work on behalf of foundations, participants help determine who receives funding. This is generally a rigorous, time-consuming, and often contentious process.[28]

STAFFING OF BIOMEDICAL RESEARCH INSTITUTIONS

Recruitment of qualified personnel is another basic activity through which a biomedical research program is organized and justified. The process may start with the selection of an individual to head the unit. Normally, the director is a senior scientist, perhaps the individual who pioneered or first achieved major successes in the chosen field of investigations. A unit has an enormous advantage if it is headed by someone knowledgeable in all aspects of operations, who is known and respected by colleagues throughout the discipline, and who commands the trust of the institution's backers. There is, however, no foregone conclusion that the most productive investigators available would be willing to assume executive command. Many capable scientists are philosophically opposed to devoting precious time and energy to administrative duties and take pains to eschew such appointments. The direction of large research organizations may, therefore, be entrusted to individuals who have chosen managerial or entrepreneurial goals over direct involvement in scientific discovery.[29]

Formal academic training is obviously a basic consideration in the recruitment of the scientific staff. A doctoral degree has long been the basic credential for employment and advancement as a full professional in biomedical research institutions. Clinical research units may require investigators to have an M.D. degree. For work in one of the basic sciences, a Ph.D. or Sc.D. degree in a relevant discipline may be preferred. Recognizing the importance of both tracks of graduate education to careers in advanced biomedical research, many institutions seek candidates with combined doctorates, particularly graduates of a recognized university Medical Science Training Program, sponsored by funds from the NIH.[30] Still more significant, however, is the reputation of the university where an individual studied, the reputation of advisors and mentors, and whether significant scientific experience was acquired through postdoctoral fellowships or residencies.[31]

The work of visiting and part-time professional staff is a significant factor at many biomedical research institutions. Researchers in these categories are often as numerous as the regular, full-time investigators. At academic medical centers, this may result from joint staff appointments to hospital services and teaching departments. Independent institutions have traditionally attracted the participation of visiting researchers during the summer, when professorial scientists are relieved of their teaching responsibilities at academic medical centers.

Various numbers of technicians, clerical staff, and other, less skilled workers are ranked below the professional investigators in the chain of command. Technicians may range from individuals knowledgeable and experienced enough to perform complicated assignments to untrained laboratory assistants hired to wash glassware and clean animal cages. Hiring, supervision, and other aspects of personnel management are major responsibilities of institutional administrations, just as in any organization, but in the case of research units employee performance evaluations are likely to focus on scientific contributions and specialized judgments that are unique to the field.

Despite obvious differences among employee classifications, it is important to observe that hierarchical ranking may not be as rigid at biomedical research units as in most health care delivery facilities and schools. Research units can be as pragmatic as industrial firms in rewarding and promoting talented individuals. Investigative experience, particularly a record of productive contributions to publishable discoveries, is what ultimately counts the most in establishing a research career. It is very common in biomedical science for research teams to recognize the contributions of junior members, and in many instances technicians have been promoted to professional status in recognition of expertise acquired on the job.

The risk of job instability due to dependence on grant or contract support is problematic for all employees of biomedical research institutions. A sudden demand for qualified personnel created when grant money becomes available may be followed by layoffs when grants lapse. Professional investigators as well as technicians are sometimes inconvenienced by short-term positions, but the former presumably have a stronger commitment to their work and ultimately a greater chance of gaining permanent employment.[32]

MANAGING LABORATORIES AND OTHER RESEARCH SETTINGS

Laboratories are the most typical settings for biomedical research. Their size, the types of equipment used, and the number of personnel employed vary to such a degree that little generalization is possible. Many kinds of analysis require close physical proximity to clinical examination rooms or operating rooms, and therefore the laboratories must be situated within a hospital or medical center. In other fields of research, investigations focus on nonliving substances, microorganisms, or laboratory animals that can be acquired and manipulated without connection to clinical activity.

The formats employed for recording and analyzing data likewise vary enormously. No single technological advance has necessarily rendered obsolete paper laboratory notebooks or clinical case files. New software products, however, are constantly being marketed to capture and manipulate raw data. For every research specialty, there is an ever expanding array of calculating, computing, monitoring, and testing equipment, all with digitalized data output. Computer graphics programs, many integrated with word-processing software, routinely record and store the graphic and tabular results of experiments or trials online.

Scientific laboratory apparatus, along with equipment for the clinical examinations that investigators may share with hospital colleagues, is usually expensive. Once acquired, it may be complicated or dangerous to operate. Interaction between investigators and manufacturers and suppliers can be complex. In fields where the research is at the cutting edge of technology, scientists themselves sometimes become inventors. This phenomenon was perhaps more pronounced in decades past, before the advent of microchip-regulated electronics. Even today, however, as consumers in the relatively tiny market for expensive machinery, major laboratories exercise the power to demand customized equipment. Proper security arrangements for hazardous and controlled substances and measures for their safe and legal disposal require sizable investments at many kinds of laboratories. Biomedical research institutions are also significant consumers of high-priced multipurpose items, such as computer hardware. Biomedical information transfer and biostatistics have become crucial services of large medical centers, demanding correspondingly large outlays for mainframe data processing equipment and network lines, not to mention the specialists to maintain and operate them.[33]

LABORATORY ANIMAL MANAGEMENT

Laboratory animal management is a significant area of specialization within biomedical research. A wide variety of animal species, from primates to *E. coli*, are used in experimentation. The archetypal research subject may be the guinea pig, although more frequent and extensive uses are made of rats and mice. Several mutant strains of rodent genera (e.g., the nude mouse) have been specially bred and marketed for laboratory purposes. The experimental use of higher animals, such as cats, dogs, and monkeys, is also widespread in nearly all disciplines. This is the most costly aspect of operations, because it requires extensive space for cages, systems for sanitary feed handling and cleaning of the pens, and the services of veterinarians.

Contemporary procedures and regulations governing animal experimentation have been profoundly affected by criticism or opposition from groups ranging from antivivisectionists to animal liberation partisans. Humane societies have worked to stiffen ordinances regulating the sale of impounded dogs and cats to laboratories and have demanded legislative or police investigation of certain research institutions. The U.S. Department of Agriculture, which is charged with enforcing animal welfare legislation, has repeatedly revised regulations concerning facilities, procedures, and oversight. Committees for the governance of animal experimentation are now mandatory. Biomedical research institutions across the country have in recent years expanded and upgraded their animal care facilities.

CONDUCTING CLINICAL TRIALS

Procedures for formal clinical trials are essential to the work of a substantial proportion of biomedical research institutions. Most often these are employed as means for studying the effectiveness of new drugs, but many other objectives are possible, including investigations of various elements significant in diet, fitness, genetic makeup, and social behavior. Depending on the nature of the study, an experimental laboratory may or may not be directly involved. Some kinds of clinical trials or aspects of large projects are entrusted to commercial testing companies. Federal regulations, however, require hiring a statistical and clerical staff trained to conduct surveys of sizable subject populations. Friedman and colleagues and Spicker have provided comprehensive definitions of clinical trials.[34] They indicate that every well-designed study requires a protocol incorporating written agreements between investigators, subjects, and a scientific group selected to monitor response variables. Each trial should be constructed as a means of grappling with a primary question for which there are reasonable expectations of verifiable conclusions. The study population is a subset of a general population defined by specific eligibility criteria, out of which the group of subjects actually studied is selected. Nearly all investigations of this sort require a control group with which the group receiving the new intervention can be compared. Proper calculation of the size of the respective groups is essential to ensure the statistical means of recognizing significant differences in the data.

Effective designs for clinical trials incorporate standard means for avoiding elements of bias. Some subjects participating in drug tests, for example, may be asked to receive the experimental substance, rather than the placebo. To allow such a choice to be made by the subject, however, could produce seriously skewed data. Minimal standards for a scientific trial, therefore, hold that it be "single blind." The researchers, for their part, usually need to demonstrate that they have not favored one group of subjects over another in administering the experimental substance. In a double-blind trial, neither subjects nor investigators know which intervention is administered. In a triple-blind study, not even the group monitoring responses is aware of each intervention assignment.

The agreements with subjects that are essential to conducting a clinical trial are supposed to follow the principle of informed consent. Research applications of informed consent developed implicitly over centuries within general medical ethical and legal precepts. They received, however, specific articulation at the Nuremberg trials, in the court's judgment against the Nazi concentration camp investigators, *United States v. Karl Brandt.* That decision remains the benchmark for mandating efforts toward free and enlightened decisions on the part of clinical research subjects.[35] Gaining informed consent from subjects of biomedical research is consequently one of the most elaborate and costly steps of a screening process. Warnings have regularly been voiced over the years that many investigators neglect their responsibilities in this matter to one degree or other.[36] The federal government has responded by issuing increasingly lengthy regulations governing these interactions. Chief among them is the mandate to establish institutional review boards or human subjects committees. In theory, institutional review boards are charged with scrutinizing research proposals for the protection of human subjects at any institution funded by the Department of Health and Human Services.[37]

In certain areas of clinical research, formal clinical trials and formal applications of informed consent do not apply. Many new surgical interventions, most pathology research, and various kinds of experimental psychiatric treatments are in this category. Some forms of clinical investigations, furthermore, are entirely retrospective, involving the study of inactive medical records. Much epidemiological research, for example, requires permission from hospital management for secondary analysis of data not originally created for general knowledge. Whatever the design and scope of the problem under investigation, some form of rigorous control is required to reach valid scientific conclusions.

PATIENT CARE IN BIOMEDICAL RESEARCH INSTITUTIONS

A prerequisite for conducting clinical trials in most instances is that a biomedical research institution offer clinical care services. Although some subjects participate in research investigations for reasons not related to their own health, substantially more are attracted after having first sought treatment as patients. This is one of several facets of the connections between hospitals and research units that were alluded to earlier in this chapter. Depending on the treatment specialty, a research institution itself may function as a hospital or may offer only outpatient services. All requirements for hospital or clinic licensing and other regulations that are discussed in Chapter 2 apply to biomedical research institutions that treat patients. Patient care services of independent biomedical research institutions are subject to the same centripetal forces of the U.S. health care system that have linked together originally autonomous hospitals as medical centers. Institutions may affiliate or merge services voluntarily to control costs or acquire new facilities. There also have been instances in which internal reorganization has been forced upon research units by third-party payers to simplify billing procedures.[38]

EDUCATIONAL ACTIVITIES OF BIOMEDICAL RESEARCH INSTITUTIONS

Biomedical research institutions also engage in educational activities, both informal and formal. Informal educational activity is necessitated by the fact that scientific investigations are highly specialized, employing sophisticated concepts and the latest equipment. The junior staff need to be educated regarding the use of equipment and handling of hazardous materials. Research units affiliated with academic medical centers and teaching hospitals may also play significant roles in formal educational programs. A unit could operate, for example, as a specially funded section of a basic science department at a medical school, with all the senior staff holding academic appointments. Students might be involved in projects in fulfillment of elective course work or perhaps as summer employees. Postdoctoral fellows render significant contributions to research programs, with their employment often underwritten by federal grants. (For further information on the role of research programs in health professionals' education, see Chapter 5.)

COMMUNICATION AND MARKETING OF BIOMEDICAL RESEARCH FINDINGS

Most biomedical research, particularly in the nonprofit sector, is intended to produce publishable findings. The quality of the publication as a rule is

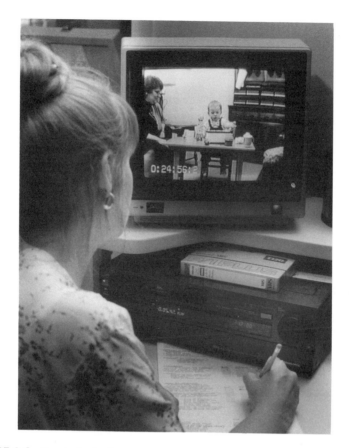

FIGURE 4–2   Psychologist Joanna Grant Nicholas studies communication skills of hearing-impaired children at Central Institute for the Deaf, St. Louis, 1993. *Source:* Central Institute for the Deaf, St. Louis, Marcus Kosa, photographer

important to investigators, and a respected refereed scientific journal is the medium of choice in most cases. The writing and editorial revision that take place before a manuscript[39] is submitted for publication are often a painstaking process. Large research institutions may employ professional writers and editors to facilitate this process. As organizational activities, such services are likely to come under administrative purview, but unlike the activities considered previously in this chapter, they are primarily focused on the end products of research rather than on beginnings.

Scientific journals in the main are published either by professional associations or by commercial firms. A significant number, however, are published directly by research institutions. An even more common variation is for a professional association to appoint an editor-in-chief and an editorial board, who then may draw on the resources of a research unit. *Neurology*, for example, the chief official organ of the American Academy of Neurology, has since its inception been edited by a series of distinguished investigators in the field, who oversee editorial operations.

An essential ingredient in editing a scientific journal is peer review of the most promising submissions. Editors normally send each manuscript to at least two experts in the field for them to judge the quality and potential of the work. Rarely do reviewers have the opportunity to test fully the methods and findings described, so their reactions are never foolproof, but overall the process provides an effective means of quality control. The identities of reviewers are generally kept confidential, and their critiques may be moderated by the editors before they render decisions about publication. The exchanges involved can be an important part of the work of a research institution.[40] (For more information on publishing in the medical field, see Chapter 7.)

Avenues of scientific communication less formal than refereed journals may also be important to research units. Bulletins and newsletters are commonly devoted to such purposes as interstaff news (a particular consideration if the unit operates in decentralized facilities or employs substantial numbers of visiting or temporary staff) and fund raising. Conferences, seminars, and symposia are frequently chosen means for disseminating information or airing common problems among colleagues. Many research institutions employ public relations personnel to tout achievements to media and directly to the general public. All these and other efforts require a significant investment of the unit's resources.

Biomedical research institutions may produce marketable inventions worth in the aggregate millions of dollars annually as products or by-products of their investigations. Certain major medical centers generate enough patentable findings to warrant hiring staffs of patent attorneys to manage the situation. This is beyond the means, however, of most smaller nonprofit institutions. Independent research units do have the option of contracting with patent management organizations, the largest of which are also equipped to handle product marketing.[41]

DOCUMENTATION OF BIOMEDICAL RESEARCH INSTITUTIONS

The work of archivists in scientific fields other than biomedicine to document what is termed "discipline history" has significant applications here. The concept of discipline history originally developed out of concern for preserving landmark records in the physical sciences and engineering. The primary goal has been to ensure adequate documentation of subject areas through joint efforts of archivists in several institutions. One of the most effective demonstrations of archival cooperation of this nature has been coordinated by the Center for the History of Physics of the American Institute of Physics (AIP) in fields such as high-energy physics, space science, and geophysics.[42]

If we ignore for a moment the obvious differences between physics and biomedicine and compare specific programs in these two disciplines, we find many similarities. Like biomedical units, institutions devoted to research in physics have many different missions and profiles, ranging from federal governmental agencies to commercial ventures. As in biomedicine, the contributions of nonprofit units are very strong. These institutions include both state-supported and private bodies, some university-affiliated, others independent. A combination of federal grant programs and private philanthropy enables them to conduct similar investigatory programs. To round out the list of similarities, much of the research performed in physics laboratories has a direct impact on biomedicine. Investigations in isotope analysis, applications of laser techniques, spectroscopy, and ultrasonics are but a few of these areas. Many examples of close collegial interaction between physicists and biomedical researchers could be cited at any large academic medical center.

THE HUMAN GENOME INITIATIVE: A MODEL SUBJECT FOR DISCIPLINE HISTORY

It is not appropriate here to discuss how receptive all research institutions in physics may be to the model established by the AIP other than to observe that it appears to work most effectively in the world of megaprojects supported primarily by governmental agencies and consortia. There are areas of biomedical research that lend themselves equally well to discipline history projects, and for similar reasons. Among the most likely current subjects is the Human Genome Project, a worldwide research effort that has the goal of mapping the entire structure of human DNA and determining the location of the estimated 100,000 human genes. Funded through the NIH and the Department of Energy, a substantial portion of the research is being conducted in the laboratories of these two agencies. In the grandest tradition of extramural programs, the NIH portion of the appropriation is shared with (at this writing) seven major centers located at universities throughout the United States. Other related program assistance is available to smaller research teams, with additional money provided for training grants, technology development, and international collaboration.[43]

The objectives of the Human Genome Project in a sense are inherently archival. This is particularly clear from one part of the NIH project, which is to establish and operate a National Center for Biotechnology Information (NCBI) within the National Library of Medicine. NCBI has the particular mission of creating automated systems for knowledge about molecular biology, biochemistry, and genetics and of pursuing research in biological information handling. NCBI is currently conducting investigations with genome research centers and libraries throughout the country about the feasibility of transmitting mapping data online. The Human Genome Project also offers opportunities for archival development through a small portion (3 percent) of the budget allocated to address ethical, legal, and social considerations. Arguing that the full implications of the project on society cannot be understood unless appropriate records on a wide range of issues are collected and retained, at least two private organizations have begun discipline history studies on genome research.[44]

Currently, the most comprehensive effort in this regard is being mounted by the Chemical Heritage Foundation, an organization sponsored by the American Chemical Society and the Society of Chemical Engineers (and openly modeled on the AIP). The CHF project, titled BIMOSI, or Biomolecular Sciences Initiative, is interested not only in genome research but in all important investigations pertaining to molecular biology. At this writing, the staff of BIMOSI have begun to advise researchers and their organizations about what to preserve and where, and how to conduct oral histories. A somewhat more limited documentation project is under way at the National Center for Bioethics Literature, of the Kennedy Institute of Ethics at Georgetown University, focusing on the ethical, legal, and social implications of human genome research. Historians and archivists involved in both projects acknowledge the enormity of their respective undertakings, in particular challenges related to the diversity of interests of individual researchers and their parent institutions.[45]

OBSTACLES TO DOCUMENTATION PLANNING FOR BIOMEDICAL RESEARCH INSTITUTIONS

The opportunity that has developed for a discipline history project on genome research is unusual among biomedical research fields. The combination of factors—novelty, urgency, international collaboration, and above all, the generous public funding of the project—is more characteristic of the great crash programs in nuclear physics than any recent field of medical investigation. It is worth examining here why there were no comparable calls for discipline history centers to address earlier national mandates for biomedical research, such as the "wars" declared on cancer from the 1930s through the 1980s.[46]

The differences are at least fourfold. First, as already noted, there is the proliferation of biomedical research institutions in the United States. Consider, for example, a hypothetical history center for cancer oncology. Counting only the units that truly specialize in problems and issues relating to malignancies, one would have to deal not with seven major centers, as with the Human Genome Project, but perhaps seven times seventy.[47] For better or worse (and certainly, in the case of cancer, there have been many arguments to the effect that the proliferation of research institutions has resulted in much duplication and waste), the extramural grant system and private philanthropy have never concentrated their funding eggs in only a few baskets.

Second, there is the general issue of confidentiality of clinical data. Essentially, this is an area governed by the same constraints involving patient records discussed in Chapter 2. Research units within hospitals and academic medical centers are required to safeguard the identities of study subjects as completely as they do the identities of regular patients. For this reason, they normally deny outside researchers (or anyone else) access to clinical data that they have generated or augmented for investigative purposes.[48]

A third difference reflects the enormous contributions of private, profit-making research institutions to every biomedical field. Competition alone dictates that information about their proprietary discoveries not be shared with other organizations or individuals, at least until the data no longer have market value. Companies that have developed new drugs for the treatment of cancer (or HIV infections, or any other focus of a health crisis) find themselves under great pressure to justify decisions about the costs, marketing, and distribution of their products. They are certain, therefore, to be armed with policies concerning what they will disseminate to the public and what they will withhold.

A fourth difference is more a matter of philosophy and custom than legal substance. This relates to the traditional reliance on refereed journals as the primary medium for reporting—and preserving the historical record of—biomedical discoveries in the academic sector. For most biomedical scientists, journals are the true archives: at best, they convey succinctly the nature of discoveries, discuss their implications, and provide necessary directions for replicating the experiments. Unlike findings from projects in sciences and technologies that are commissioned for national security operations or commercial enterprises, most investigations in medicine and allied fields are intended to produce publishable results. Despite fierce competition among scientists for the attention of editors and review panels of the most respected journals, findings of most reputable health science projects appear sooner or later in print.[49] It is no accident that the titles of well over one hundred biomedical serial publications representing a wide range of investigative fields begin with variations of the term "archives."

The narrow implication of this tradition is that special repositories for original research data are unnecessary. Several indications, however, point to a greater realization within the biomedical research community than in the past that measures must be taken to preserve documentation generated by significant projects. Hedrick in 1985 offered an extensive summary of these issues.[50] They include wider opportunities for verification, refutation, or refinement of original results; the chance for replications with multiple data sets; encouragement of new questions and multiple perspectives employing the original data; the creation of new data sets through data file linkages; reductions in the incidence of faked and inaccurate results; dissemination of knowledge about analytic techniques and research designs; and the provision of expanded resources for training of future scientists. Other authors address the possibility that some researchers who have been supported by public funding may be compelled to preserve and share their data with others.[51]

CURRENT ARCHIVAL COVERAGE OF BIOMEDICAL RESEARCH INSTITUTIONS

Archival repositories located throughout the United States hold extensive records of biomedical research. These records, however, almost exclusively pertain to scientific investigations conducted at hospitals, federal government–operated laboratories, and educational institutions. (See Chapters 2, 3, and 5 for examples of major collections in these respective categories.) Documentation of the functions of specialized biomedical research units, by contrast, is located in relatively few repositories. Instances mainly reflect the academic connections of the principal investigators; an example is papers of distinguished scientists preserved in university archives. Individual prominence has also led to the placement of relevant collections in certain general repositories, among them the Library of Congress, the National Library of Medicine, the Smithsonian Institution, the American Philosophical Library (Philadelphia), and the State Historical Society of Wisconsin (Madison). The records of the General Education Board of the Rockefeller Foundation in the Rockefeller Archive Center are important for their coverage of early twentieth-century foundation support of biomedical research institutions. Rarely has an independent nonprofit institution in the fields examined here established its own archives, as is the case with the Cold Spring Harbor Laboratory. The commitment to archives or discipline history on the part of specialty profit-making biomedical research enterprises is, at this writing, an unknown. A patient, persistent, and long-term investigation by a discipline history group dedicated to biomedical research, along the lines of the AIP or the Chemical Heritage Foundation, could yield important information.[52]

NOTES

1. Various directories of biomedical research organizations follow significantly different criteria in the selection and arrangement of their listings. The *Encyclopedia of Medical Organizations and Agencies (EMOA)*, 3rd ed. (Detroit: Gale Research, 1990), for example, lists more than 2,500 research organizations, including approximately 700 U.S. government research centers and programs and approximately 1,800 university-related and other nonprofit institutions outside of federal agencies. Entries in *EMOA* are divided into 69 biomedical specialty areas, all but two of which are the focus of at least one research center in the United States. The *Research Centers Directory (RCD,)* 16th ed. (Detroit: Gale Research, 1991) covers university research centers and other nonprofit research organizations in both the United States and Canada but does not list the federal government agencies of either country. "Medical and Health Sciences," the third of seventeen sections, contains almost 2,000 entries. An additional 1,000 institutions that are devoted to the basic biomedical and behavioral sciences may be found listed in three other sections of *RCD*. Commercial research institutions in the United States, which do not appear in either of the publications just mentioned, account for about 1,800 of the entries in *The Biotechnology Directory* (1991 ed., J. Coombs and Y. R. Alston, New York: Stockton Press, 1990).
2. Donald S. Fredrickson, "Biomedical Research in the 1980s," *New England Journal of Medicine* 304 (1981): 513.
3. Biomedical research institutions in these respects are typical of a much larger web of institutions that cut across government, nonprofit, and industrial lines. See Louis Galambos and Joseph Pratt, *The Rise of the Corporate Commonwealth: U.S. Business and Public Policy in the Twentieth Century* (New York: Basic Books, 1988), and Louis Galambos, ed., *The New American State: Bureaucracies and Policies Since World War II* (Baltimore: Johns Hopkins University Press, 1987).
4. Robert Q. Marston, "Influence of NIH Policy Past and Present on the University Health Education Complex," in H. Hugh Fudenberg and Vijaya L. Melnick, eds., *Biomedical Scientists and Public Policy* (New York: Plenum Press, 1978); Robert J. Glaser, "The Impact of Philanthropy on Medicine and Health," *Perspectives in Biology and Medicine* 36 (1992): 46–56; and George F. Cahill, "The Role of Foundations in the Future of Medicine," *Clinical and Investigative Medicine* 9, no.4 (1986): 273–77.
5. Internal Revenue Code 170A-9(b)(1)(iii).

6. Barbara J. Kirschten, "Obtaining Tax-Exempt Status for Medical Research Organizations," *Tax Management, Estates, Gifts, and Trusts Journal* 15 (1990): 28–32.
7. Internal Revenue Code 170A-9(b)(1)(ii).
8. For official listings and program statements, see *The United State Government Manual* (Office of the Federal Register, National Archives and Records Administration, annual). See also Alice K. Dustira, "The Funding of Basic and Clinical Biomedical Research," in Roger J. Porter and Thomas E. Malone, eds., *Biomedical Research: Collaboration and Conflict of Interest* (Baltimore: Johns Hopkins University Press, 1992), 33–56.
9. Arthur Kornberg, *For the Love of Enzymes: The Odyssey of a Biochemist* (Cambridge: Harvard University Press, 1989), 1–8, 29–31, 79–83, 121–34.
10. Information drawn in part from an information bulletin, "Mayo Graduate School of Medicine . . . Postdoctoral Research Fellowship Programs" (Mayo Clinic and Foundation, Rochester, Minn., 1991).
11. Rosemary Stevens, *In Sickness and in Wealth: American Hospitals in the Twentieth Century* (New York: Basic Books, 1989). For more information on academic health centers, see Joan D. Krizack, "The Context for Documentation Planning in Academic Health Centers," in Nancy McCall and Lisa A. Mix, eds., *Designing Archival Programs to Advance Knowledge in the Health Fields* (Baltimore: Johns Hopkins University Press, 1994).
12. Christopher C. Vaughn et al., "The Contribution of Biomedical Sciences and Technology to U.S. Economic Competitiveness," in Porter and Malone, *Biomedical Research*, 57–76.
13. Wayne Biddle, "A Patent on Knowledge: Harvard Goes Public," *Harper's*, July 1981, 22–26, and Bernard D. Reams, *University-Industry Research Partnerships* (Westport, Conn.: Quorum Books, 1986), 105.
14. Paul G. Waugaman and Roger J. Porter, "Mechanisms of Interactions between Industry and the Academic Medical Center," in Porter and Malone, *Biomedical Research*, 93–118.
15. Reams, *University-Industry Research Partnerships*, 105–326, devotes extensive coverage to selected contracts.
16. Waugaman and Porter, "Mechanisms of Interactions," 111–14.
17. Richard S. Ross, "Academic Research and Industry Relationships," *Clinical and Investigative Medicine* 9 (1986): 268–72, and Thomas W. Langfitt et al., eds., *Partners in the Research Enterprise: University-Corporate Relations in Science and Technology* (Philadelphia: University of Pennsylvania Press, 1983).
18. Reams, *University-Industry Research Partnerships*, 123–24, 146.
19. Joan K[rizack] Haas, Helen Willa Samuels, and Barbara Trippel Simmons, *Appraising the Records of Modern Science and Technology: A Guide* (Cambridge: Massachusetts Institute of Technology, 1985), although not addressing biomedical research directly, is a substantial guide to understanding the process and stages of scientific investigations. See especially the Table of Scientific and Technological Activities and Their Records, 20.
20. Howard H. Hiatt, *America's Health in the Balance: Choice or Chance?* (New York: Harper & Row, 1987), 156–61, and William Paton, *Man and Mouse: Animals in*

Medical Research (New York: Oxford University Press, 1984), 23–24. Bioethicists in particular draw distinctions between therapeutic and nontherapeutic research (or between validated and nonvalidated practices). See Thomas A. Mappes and Jane S. Zembaty, *Biomedical Ethics*, 3rd ed. (New York: McGraw-Hill, 1991), 204–9. For the concept of clinical research placed into international perspective, see Jacques Genest, "Modern Concept of the Organization of Clinical Research," *Clinical and Investigative Medicine* 9 (1986): 256–60.

21. Quoted by James B. Wyngaarden in "The Role of Government Support in Biomedical Research," *Clinical and Investigative Medicine* 9 (1986): 265–68.
22. Washington University, Division of Biology and Biomedical Sciences, *Faculty Research* (catalog), 1992–1993, 1992.
23. For a broad archival survey of industries of the kind involved here, see Bruce H. Bruemmer and Sheldon Hochheiser, *The High-Technology Company: A Historical Research and Archival Guide* (Minneapolis: Charles Babbage Institute, University of Minnesota, 1989).
24. Michael Spector, "The Case of Dr. Gallo," *New York Review of Books*, 15 Aug. 1991, 52.
25. Robert F. Jones, *American Medical Education: Institutions, Programs, and Issues* (Washington, D.C.: Association of American Medical Colleges, 1992), 21.
26. Gerald F. Anderson and Catherine M. Russe, "Biomedical Research and Technology Development," *Health Affairs* 6 (1987): 85–92.
27. Jones, *American Medical Education*, 22.
28. Philip Abelson, "Mechanisms for Evaluating Scientific Information and the Role of Peer Review," *Journal of the American Society for Information Science* 41 (1990): 216–22, and Susan Crawford, Loretta Stucki, "Peer Review and the Changing Research Record," ibid., 223–28.
29. Virginia P. White, *Handbook of Research Laboratory Management* (Philadelphia: ISI Press, 1988), 18–20.
30. Carl Frieden and Barbara J. Fox, "Career Choices of Graduates from Washington University's Medical Scientist Training Program," *Academic Medicine* 66, no.3 (1991): 162–64.
31. White, *Research Laboratory Management*, 46–58.
32. Waneta C. Tuttle et al., "Considerations of Managing Large-Scale Clinical Trials," *Journal of the Society of Research Administrators* 21, no.2 (1989): 13–22.
33. It does not always follow that well-funded investigations use the best equipment. A National Science Foundation study in the early 1980s revealed that less than 20 percent of existing apparatus used in academic research in the biological and medical sciences was state of the art. Many buildings and laboratory facilities erected in the early days of NIH funding (the late 1940s to the early 1960s), moreover, urgently need modernization. See E. Jill Hurt, ed., *Health Policy Agenda for the American People* (Chicago: Health Policy Agenda for the American People, 1987), 2: 157.
34. Laurence M. Friedman, Curt D. Furberg, and David L. DeMets, *Fundamentals of Clinical Trials* (Littleton, Mass.: PSG, 1985); Stuart F. Spicker, *The Use of*

Human Beings in Research: With Special Reference to Clinical Trials (Boston:
Kluwer, 1988); and Tuttle et al., "Large-Scale Clinical Trials."
35. Paul Appelbaum, Charles W. Lidz, and Alan Meisel, *Informed Consent: Legal Theory and Clinical Practice* (New York: Oxford University Press, 1987), 211–19; Ruth Faden, Tom L. Beauchamp, and Nancy M. P. King, *A History and Theory of Informed Consent* (New York: Oxford University Press, 1986), 151–87; and David J. Rothman, *Strangers at the Bedside: A History of How Law and Bioethics Transformed Medical Decision Making* (New York: Basic Books, 1991).
36. David L. Wheeler, "Informed Consent Questioned in Research Using Humans," *Chronicle of Higher Education*, 4 Dec. 1991, A14.
37. Code of Federal Regulations, Title 45, pt. 46, Protection of Human Subjects, revised March 8, 1983. The portions of the Code that specify how institutional review boards (IRBs) are to be established and operated include the following: "Each IRB shall have at least five members, with varying backgrounds to promote complete and adequate review of research activities commonly conducted by the institution. The IRB shall be sufficiently qualified through the experience and expertise of its members, and the diversity of the members' backgrounds including consideration of the racial and cultural backgrounds of members and sensitivity to such issues as community attitudes, to promote respect for its advice and counsel in safeguarding the rights and welfare of human subjects." A subsequent part of the same section of the regulation indicates that each IRB shall include "at least one member whose primary concerns are in nonscientific areas (45 CFR 46.107)." See also Applebaum et al., *Informed Consent*, 219–28.
38. Two institutions at the Washington University Medical Center illustrate situations of this nature: Barnard Free Skin and Cancer Hospital, a research hospital in St. Louis that was originally independent, merged with the university in 1950 and lost its autonomy in patient care four years later, when it moved to the medical center campus. Barnard now functions as an endowed research and treatment program of the university medical school and Barnes Hospital, the center's principal teaching hospital. In 1992, Mallinckrodt Institute of Radiology, the clinical treatment arm of the university's radiology department, transferred most of its patient services at Barnes Hospital to the hospital administration in the interests of simplifying billing procedures, as required by Medicare and commercial insurers.
39. Archival readers are advised that the research world ineluctably uses the term *manuscript* almost exclusively in this context.
40. Arnold S. Relman, "Medical Research, Medical Journals, and the Public Interest," *Journal of the Society of Research Administrators* 21, no.2 (1989): 7–12; Abelson, "Evaluating Scientific Information"; and Crawford and Stucki, "Peer Review."
41. White, 1988, 140–47.
42. Joan Warnow-Blewett, "Saving the Records of Science and Technology: The Role of a Discipline History Center," *Science and Technology Libraries* 7 (1987): 29–40; "The Role of a Discipline History Center, Part II: Promoting Archives

and Research in Science and Technology," *Science and Technology Libraries* 9 (1988–89): 85–102. See also AIP, *AIP Study of Multi-Institutional Collaborations: Phase I: High Energy Physics* (New York: AIP, Center for History of Physics, 1992) issues of the *AIP History Newsletter*, 1989-present, that describe a long-term study of interinstitutional collaborations in physics and allied sciences.

43. U.S. Department of Health and Human Services, U.S. Department of Energy, *Understanding Our Genetic Inheritance, the U.S. Human Genome Project: The First Five Years, FY 1991–1995* (Washington, D.C.: Government Printing Office, 1990); and John Beatty and Elizabeth E. Sandager, "Documenting the Human Genome Project: Challenges and Opportunities," draft report, History of Science Society, 1992.

44. U.S. Department of Health and Human Services, *Understanding Our Genetic Inheritance*, and unpublished communication with David Lipman, NCBI, and Susan Crawford, Washington University School of Medicine Library.

45. The Chemical Heritage Society publishes a quarterly newsletter, *Chemical Heritage* (formerly *The Beckman Center for Chemistry News*); unpublished communication with Susan Lindee and Elizabeth E. Sandager, Chemical Heritage Foundation; Doris Mueller Goldstein, National Reference Center for Bioethics Literature, Georgetown University, 1990–1991; Elizabeth E. Sandager, "Report on Los Alamos Exploratory Site Visit," on behalf of the Chemical Heritage Foundation, unpublished, 1992. Other prominent efforts to document the human genome project are led and coordinated by Victoria A. Harden of the NIH Historical office.

46. For a comprehensive account of the "cancer wars," see James T. Patterson, *The Dread Disease: Cancer and Modern American Culture* (Cambridge: Harvard University Press, 1987).

47. The actual total, suggested by *EMOA* and *RCD*, would fall between 400 and 500.

48. Brian Jay Yolles, Joseph C. Connors, and Seymour Grufferman, "Obtaining Access to Data from Government-Sponsored Medical Research," *New England Journal of Medicine* 315 (1986): 1669–72.

49. Relman, "Medical Research, Medical Journals, and the Public Interest."

50. Terry E. Hedrick, "Justifications for and Obstacles to Data Sharing," in Stephen E. Fienberg, Margaret E. Martin, and Miron L. Straf, eds., *Sharing Research Data* (Washington, D.C.: National Academy Press, 1985), 123–47. See also Jane Williams, "The Importance of Preserving Scientific Data," in McCall and Mix, eds., *Designing Archival Programs*.

51. Joe Shelby Cecil and Eugene Griffin, "The Role of Legal Policies in Data Sharing," in Fienberg et al., *Sharing Research Data*; Cecil and Robert Boruch, "Compelled Disclosure of Research Data: An Early Warning and Suggestions for Psychologists," *Law and Human Behavior* 12 (1988): 181–89; and Yolles et al., "Obtaining Access to Data."

52. David Bearman and John T. Edsall, eds., *Archival Sources of the History of Biochemistry and Molecular Biology: A Reference Guide and Report* (Boston: American Academy of Arts and Sciences, 1980), is still the most complete guide to existing archival collections from biomedical research institutions.

SELECT ANNOTATED BIBLIOGRAPHY

Abelson, Philip. "Mechanisms for Evaluating Scientific Information and the Role of Peer Review." *Journal of the American Society for Information Science* 41 (1990): 216–22. Examines the effects of the "publish or perish" syndrome on research publication and discounts reports of widespread fraud.

American Institute of Physics, Center for History of Physics. *AIP Study of Multi-Institutional Collaborations, Phase I: High-Energy Physics.* New York: American Institute of Physics, 1992. An enormously valuable model for any scientific discipline history project; divided into reports (no. 1: "Summary and Recommendations"; no. 2: "Documenting Collaborations"; no. 3: "Catalog of Selected Historical Materials") by various authors, principally Joan Warnow-Blewett (see also below).

Bearman, David, and John T. Edsall, eds. *Archival Sources of the History of Biochemistry and Molecular Biology: A Reference Guide and Report.* Boston: American Academy of Arts and Sciences, 1980. A classic survey of archival holdings in key biomedical sciences.

Bruemmer, Bruce H., and Sheldon Hochheiser. *The High-Technology Company: A Historical Research and Archival Guide.* Minneapolis: Charles Babbage Institute, University of Minnesota, 1989. Describes the research function and its activities in high-technology companies.

Cahill, George F. "The Role of Foundations in the Future of Medicine." *Clinical and Investigative Medicine* 9, no.4 (1986): 273–77. Sees a slow decline in philanthropic support for biomedical research, made up in part by academic-private sector contracts.

Frederickson, Donald S. "Biomedical Research in the 1980s." *New England Journal of Medicine* 304 (1981): 509–17. The title notwithstanding, a good short history of biomedical research before the decade began.

Friedman, Lawrence M., et al. *Fundamentals of Clinical Trials,* 2nd ed. Littleton, Mass.: PSG Publishing Co., 1985. A comprehensive and clearly written introduction to a basic methodology.

Fudenberg, H. Hugh, and Vjaya L. Melnick, eds. *Biomedical Scientists and Public Policy.* New York: Plenum Press, 1978. A collection of essays on problems and issues in public funding of research.

Haas, Joan K[rizack], Helen Willa Samuels, and Barbara Trippel Simmons. *Appraising the Records of Modern Science and Technology: A Guide.* Boston: Massachusetts Institute of Technology, 1985. An overview of documentation generated in the various stages of scientific and technological research (although, with few specific references to biomedicine); well organized and illustrated.

Hedrick, Terry E. "Justifications for and Obstacles to Data Sharing." In *Sharing Research Data,* edited by Stephen E. Fienberg, Margaret E. Martin, and Miron L. Straf. Washington, D.C.: National Academy Press, 1985. Finds little reliable information about scientific data sharing; advocates careful cost-benefit analysis.

Hiatt, Howard H. *America's Health in the Balance: Choice or Chance?* New York:

Harper & Row, 1987. Chapter 10, "Biomedical Research," advocates taxing all health-related goods and services to fund scientific investigations.

Institute of Medicine, Division of Health Sciences Policy, Committee on the Responsible Conduct of Research. *The Responsible Conduct of Research in the Health Sciences.* Washington, D.C.: National Academy Press, 1989. Examines issues related to biomedical research fraud; proposes ways of encouraging ethical standards without stifling research freedom and creativity.

Langfitt, Thomas W., et al., eds. *Partners in the Research Enterprise: University-Corporate Relations in Science and Technology.* Philadelphia: University of Pennsylvania Press, 1983. Proceedings of a national conference on university-corporate relations in science and technology held at the University of Pennsylvania in 1982.

Porter, Roger J., and Thomas E. Malone, eds. *Biomedical Research: Collaboration and Conflict of Interest.* Baltimore: Johns Hopkins University Press, 1992. Analyzes problems of biomedical research funding, especially academic-industrial partnerships, from a university perspective.

Reams, Bernard D. *University-Industry Research Partnerships.* Westport, Conn.: Quorum Books, 1986. An extensive historical and legal analysis, illustrated by appendices containing the texts of four landmark contracts, three of which concern biomedical research.

Relman, Arnold S. "Medical Research, Medical Journals, and the Public Interest." *Journal of the Society of Research Administrators* 21 (1989): 7–12. The former editor of the *New England Journal of Medicine* discusses the mechanics of peer-reviewed journals and argues that most substantive findings in biomedical research are published.

———."What Is Clinical Research?" *Clinical Research* 9, no. 3 (1961): 516–18. A brief historical review.

Ross, Richard S. "Academic Research and Industry Relationships." *Clinical and Investigative Medicine* 9, no. 4 (1986): 269–72. Argues that, overall, academic-industrial partnerships are worth the risks.

Rothman, David J. *Strangers at the Bedside: A History of How Law and Bioethics Transformed Medical Decision Making.* New York: Basic Books, 1991. Chapter 5, "New Rules for the Laboratory," explores problems in research ethics, especially involving human subjects, and bureaucratic responses from the NIH and the Food and Drug Administration.

Strickland, Stephen P. *The Story of the NIH Grants Programs.* Lanham, Md.: University Press of America, 1988. A short monograph in eleven chapters, covering developments from Public Health Service–funded research in the 1930s to NIH's growing pains of the later 1960s, with a few cursory glances at events since then.

Swann, John P. *Academic Scientists and the Pharmaceutical Industry: Cooperative Research in Twentieth-Century America.* Baltimore: Johns Hopkins University Press, 1988. Traces cooperative biomedical research partnerships between universities and industry back to the 1920s; includes classic case studies, such as the collaboration of the Banting group at the University of Toronto with Eli Lilly in the discovery of insulin.

Warnow-Blewett, Joan. "Saving the Records of Science and Technology: The Role of a Discipline History Center." *Science and Technology Libraries* 7 (1987): 29–40; "The Role of a Discipline History Center, Part II: Promoting Archives and Research in Science and Technology." Ibid. 9 (1988–89): 85–101. These articles discuss the development of programs at the Center for the History of Physics of the American Institute of Physics, especially strategies for selection and archival placement of key research documentation. (See also citation under American Institute of Physics.)

Wyngaarden, James B. "The Role of Government Support in Biomedical Research." *Clinical and Investigative Medicine* 9, no. 4 (1986): 265–68. A brief sketch of the "panorama of national support for health research and development in the United States."

CHAPTER 5

Educational Institutions and Programs for Health Occupations

NANCY McCALL AND LISA A. MIX

OVERVIEW OF INSTRUCTIONAL PROGRAMS IN THE HEALTH FIELDS

A broad range of instructional programs provide students with the requisite knowledge, skills and credentials for occupations in the health fields. Academic preparation for these occupations is designed to instill in students specialized knowledge, problem-solving skills, and responsible modes of professional conduct. The functions of these instructional programs are, therefore, to provide intellectual, technical, and practical training of the various disciplines.[1] Although the programs focus on tradition and established standards, they are not immutable. Each generation of graduates brings a cycle of change through fresh insights and new approaches to their respective professions.

Instructional programs for occupations in the health fields occupy a unique place in the U.S. educational system. Whereas the controls for most instructional programs for other occupations are determined largely by the institutions in which they are based, the controls for instructional programs in the health fields are almost always defined outside their immediate institutional setting. Because most institutional programs in the health fields interface with practical training that involves patients and human subjects, they are more tightly controlled by legislative bodies (both state and national) and voluntary and professional associations. Institutions with instructional programs for occupations in the health fields must comply with a vast and complex array of external legislation, regulatory requirements, and professional standards of various disciplines in the health professions and related sciences and also the biological sciences/life sciences.

Because these outside controls change frequently and rapidly to accommodate new developments in the health fields, they bring regular and fast-paced change to instructional programs for health-related occupations. Because instructional programs in the arts and humanities and other related fields have fewer outside controls, they usually are not compelled to adopt uniform requirements, revise curriculum, or reform standards as often as instructional programs in the health fields. As a result, the core requirements for instructional programs in these other fields tend to vary on a national basis from institution to institution. By contrast, the core requirements for instructional programs in the health fields have greater uniformity throughout the country from institution to institution. Because of the many external pressures to keep current, instructional programs in the health fields are among the most pro-active and highly energized programs in American higher education.

Instruction for occupations in the health fields occurs mainly in two types of institutional setting[2]: educational institutions (colleges, universities, and postsecondary vocational institutions) and health care delivery facilities. In many cases, reciprocal arrangements exist between these two types of institution. In the instance of instructional programs that are based at educational institutions, a significant portion of the clinical teaching and training usually occurs in health care delivery facilities. However, much of the teaching activities of instructional programs that are based in health care delivery facilities are conducted at these institutions. Usually, the faculty for these programs are from an affiliated educational institution. These joint programs entail considerable administrative cooperation, both formal and informal. Because the records of these types of program span two or more institutional settings, archivists from the institutions involved should be prepared to collaborate in their documentation planning efforts. Major sites that combine institutions of higher education with health care delivery facilities are known as academic medical centers or academic health centers. At these centers the functions of health care delivery, education, and research are highly integrated. In some instances interinstitutional archival programs have been established at academic medical centers. For example, the archives of the Johns Hopkins Medical Institutions encompass the university health divisions (School of Medicine, University School of Nursing, School of Hygiene and Public Health, Welch Medical Library) and the Johns Hopkins Hospital.

Educational degree programs and training certificate programs are the two basic program tracks in the health fields. Degree programs are based largely in educational institutions with practical training components in health care delivery facilities. Training certificate programs may be based in either educational institutions or health care delivery facilities. Certificate programs in educational institutions are usually affiliated with health care delivery facilities, enabling students to receive practical training.

Degree programs are more comprehensive in terms of the amount of intellectual preparation and extent of practical training than certificate programs; they take longer for students to complete and are more costly for institutions to run. The fee for tuition in degree programs is generally significantly higher than in certificate programs.[3] However, the high tuition costs of professional degree programs usually yield greater long-term returns because graduates of these programs generally attain the most autonomous and highly paid occupations in the U.S. health care system, while graduates of certificate programs are usually limited to subsidiary and lower-paid occupations.

Because most degree and certificate programs for occupations in the health fields require both theoretical study and practical training, they are most often conducted in dual settings—in educational institutions and in health care delivery facilities. Theoretical studies are usually conducted at educational institutions, while supervised practical training is held at health care delivery facilities.

The practical training component is an especially critical part of academic preparation for the health occupations. Learning how to perform many clinical and technical applications can only be accomplished through the practice of doing. The experience of practical training also affords students opportunities to apply problem-solving skills by confronting the uncertainties of clinical practice in a supervised setting. Thus, in the health fields learning by doing brings the concept of practice to the formalism of higher education.

Instructional programs for occupations in the health fields are stringently regulated and highly standardized at the program level rather than at the institutional level. External forces from the public and private sectors play a greater role than institutional policy in determining the scope and standards of these programs. Professional educational and health care associations in the private sector usually take the lead in setting program standards and codes of professional conduct; legislative bodies and governmental agencies, however, are primarily responsible for adopting laws and regulations and for monitoring compliance to them. The regulatory controls for instructional programs in the health fields frequently contain special implications for archivists. Often they include stipulations about the management and preservation of particular documentation. Although a central administration division such as the registrar's office or academic affairs section usually administers institutional compliance with external regulatory controls, archivists frequently bear responsibilities for managing the long-term retention and use of this documentation. As part of their documentation planning efforts for instructional programs in the health fields, archivists need to work carefully with registrars or other appropriate administrators to identify the documentation that must be designated for long-term preservation. Documentation of the credentials earned by students at these institutions is of particular importance.

A symbiotic relationship exists between these instructional programs and current needs in the health fields. As requirements for occupational practice change, corresponding changes are usually also made in the curriculum of the programs. For instance as the Clinton administration presses for more general practitioners, medical schools are re-assessing their curriculum with this in mind. Many of the same professional associations, governmental agencies, and legislative bodies that regulate occupational practices in the health fields also regulate the instructional programs for these occupations. These external controls function as a means of compelling the programs to keep pace with change. The literature published by the professional associations and governmental agencies that regulate occupations and instructional programs in the health fields is an especially useful information resource for archivists. As a rule, it provides specific details about program and occupational requirements at the same time it presents an overview of the intellectual and technical scope of the programs and occupations.

Because instructional programs in the health fields must constantly revise and upgrade curricula and standards, they are among the most forward-looking and innovative programs in postsecondary education. They are incubators for new ideas in education as well as in health care delivery and research. Much basic research in the health, life, and biological sciences is conducted in conjunction with instructional programs, and the programs are often testing grounds for new policies, practices, and materials in the health fields.

TYPES OF INSTITUTION WITH INSTRUCTIONAL PROGRAMS FOR OCCUPATIONS IN THE U.S. HEALTH CARE SYSTEM

The types of educational and training institution for occupations in the U.S. health care system are as varied as the occupations that are part of it. The two major types of institution, educational institutions and health care delivery facilities, can be broken down into the following categories:

Educational Institutions
- Universities
- Colleges (two-year and four-year)
- Vocational and technical schools

Health Care Delivery Facilities
- Hospitals
- Others (e.g., hospices, health maintenance organizations, nursing homes)

EDUCATIONAL INSTITUTIONS

Instruction for health care occupations takes place in most types of institutions of higher education, as well as in vocational and technical institutions. *Universities* generally offer a broad range of programs, through the doctoral degree in varying configurations of professional and research fields; most universities give high priority to research. *Colleges* offer associate and baccalaureate degrees in the liberal arts or occupational fields; many two-year colleges provide a variety of certificate programs, and four-year colleges often conduct master's degree programs in such fields as nursing. *Vocational and technical schools* offer certificate programs and, in some cases, associate of arts degrees, leading to employment in the ancillary health care occupations.

Educational institutions with instructional programs for the health care professions fall into two broad groups: general educational institutions with specialized programs for the health occupations, and specialized institutions geared specifically to instruction in health care occupations. The most comprehensive example of a general educational institution is a university. Universities may administer any combination of professional schools (such as schools of medicine, nursing, public health, veterinary medicine, and dentistry), graduate and undergraduate degree programs, and paraprofessional training programs. Colleges are also general educational institutions that have instructional programs for health care occupations. Thus, archivists of many educational institutions are responsible for the records of instructional programs for health care occupations. The records of some publicly supported educational institutions, however, are sometimes under the jurisdiction of public archives.

Educational and training institutions that specialize in the health care occupations include junior colleges, professional schools, and vocational and technical schools. The Central Maine Medical Center School of Nursing and the Forsyth School for Dental Hygienists in Massachusetts are examples of two-year colleges that train students specifically for health care occupations. Professional schools in chiropractic, nursing, pharmacy, and optometry, as well as a few medical schools, exist as freestanding professional schools or specialized institutions. Meharry Medical College and the Philadelphia College of Osteopathic Medicine are examples of freestanding medical schools and medical centers; the Massachusetts College of Pharmacy and Allied Health Sciences and the Southern College of Optometry are examples of schools for related and ancillary health occupations; and the National Education Center, with locations around the country, is an example of a vocational/technical school.

HEALTH CARE DELIVERY FACILITIES

Although their primary function is patient care, hospitals, and to a lesser extent other health care delivery facilities, also play an important role in educating individuals for occupations in the health fields. Some instructional programs for nurses, physician assistants, and technicians are hospital-based. Medical internship and residency programs are usually administered by hospitals, although the physicians in charge of those programs are members of the medical school faculty. Most programs based in institutions of higher education, such as those for medicine, nursing, and physical therapy, include clinical experience in a hospital, clinic, or ambulatory care facility. The parts of the curriculum that provide clinical experience for medical students are referred to as clinical clerkships. Hospices, nursing homes, and health maintenance organizations also serve as sites for students' practical experience. Although these other health care delivery facilities have traditionally played a lesser role than hospitals in training health care professionals, the trend is beginning to reverse.

Administrative relationships between educational or training institutions and health care delivery facilities vary. The Council of Teaching Hospitals identifies three levels of affiliation between hospitals and medical schools. *Graduate* indicates that the hospital is used by the school for graduate training programs only (i.e., for interns, residents, and fellows who have completed the M.D. degree). *Major* affiliation signifies that the hospital is an important part of the teaching program of the medical school, is a major unit in the clinical clerkship program for medical students, and participates in any graduate medical education program of the medical school. *Limited* affiliation with a medical school indicates that the hospital is used in the school's teaching program only to a limited extent.[4] Almost all limited affiliations are for instructing residents and fellows only. Most medical schools have a major affiliation with one teaching hospital and have graduate or limited affiliation with other hospitals. Table 5–1 shows the intersection of institutions and degree programs.

TABLE 5–1 Institutions that conduct instructional programs for occupations in the health fields

Type of Degree or Certificate	Institutions with Degree or Certificate Programs				
	Educational Institutions			Health Care Delivery Facilities	
	Universities	Colleges	Vocational and Technical Schools	Hospitals	Other (HMOs, Nursing Homes)
Doctoral degrees	D/C			CP	CP
Masters' degrees	D/C			CP	CP
Bachelors' degrees	D/C	D/C		CP	CP
Associates' degrees		D/C	D/C	CP, D/C	CP
Postsecondary certificates	D/C	D/C	D/C	CP, D/C	CP

Abbreviations: D/C, degree or certificate; CP, clinical placement.

HISTORICAL PERSPECTIVE

THE INSTITUTIONALIZATION OF EDUCATION IN THE HEALTH FIELDS

The institutionalization of education and training for occupations in the health fields is a relatively recent phenomenon. For centuries, individual apprenticeship was the primary means of preparation for these occupations. In the United States during the eighteenth and nineteenth centuries the process of apprenticeship was gradually formalized under the aegis of special courses and placed in institutional settings, mainly hospitals and educational institutions. Preparation for the health occupations thus entered the realm of higher education.

For most of the nineteenth century, medical, dental, pharmacy, and veterinary schools were proprietary institutions that emphasized the practical elements of their professions. The faculty mainly included community practitioners whose teaching activities were secondary to their practices. Teaching consisted for the most part of lectures to large numbers of students.[5]

As progressive new approaches to teaching and research in medicine and the biological sciences evolved in Europe, many American medical students and physicians traveled to European universities and research institutes to study. When they returned, they brought a spirit of reform and new ideas. Many of these European-trained physicians joined the faculties of the leading medical schools and led the revision of curriculum to incorporate more laboratory instruction, direct participation of students in patient care under faculty supervision, and the teaching of new discoveries in bacteriology and other medical sciences. The widespread publicity given to medical advances and discoveries in bacteriology made medical students eager to learn about them. Popular demand for the most current medical knowledge in conjunction with the introduction of higher educational standards gradually forced all medical schools either to adopt curriculum reform or be faced with closure owing to declining enrollments and rising expenses.[6]

Despite the promising beginning of nursing education with the introduction of the Nightingale model, the rigor of the nursing curriculum declined as hospitals assumed control of nursing schools. In hospital-based schools the service needs of the hospital frequently took precedence over formalized studies. In many instances nursing students became little more than a source of cheap labor for the hospitals in which their schools were based.[7]

The introduction of European teaching models eventually helped to raise the quality of medical, dental, pharmacy, and veterinary education in the United States during the ninteenth century. The trend toward formalizing education in these fields was further enhanced at the turn of the century. Various legislative movements that were directed toward establishing more rigorous standards for health care practice sprang up at both the state and national levels. The passage of new laws and regulations covering practice in health care had great impact on instructional programs.[8]

Hospitals, schools, colleges, and universities were compelled to improve instructional programs to prepare students for licensing and certification procedures. Institutions that produced poorly prepared graduates who failed to obtain a license or certification for practice were eventually affected economically by the loss of students. These institutions either had to close or radically revise their educational and training procedures to meet changing standards because prospective practitioners sought to attend institutions that would best prepare them for licensing and board certification. The tightening of licensing and certification procedures eventually made the educational and training process much more competitive.

Authority over professional education gradually passed to the professional societies. For example, the Council on Medical Education of the American Medical Association (AMA) began to accredit medical schools in 1905. Subsequently, most states began to restrict licensure to practice medicine to graduates of AMA-accredited schools. The council gradually raised the standards for accreditation, which contributed to the drop in the number of medical schools from over 160 in 1900 to 86 in 1920.[9]

The medical department of the College of Philadelphia was the first American medical school to be established. Founded in 1765, it was based largely on the model of the University of Edinburgh.[10] In 1821 the first American school of pharmacy, the Philadelphia College of Pharmacy, was founded.[11] Formalized, institution-based dental education also had its beginnings in the early part of the nineteenth century. In 1825 the first dental school in North America was established in Bainbridge, Ohio; however, the Baltimore College of Dental Surgery, which opened in 1840, actually was the prototype for dental education in the United States.[12] In 1855 the Boston Veterinary Institute, the first veterinary college, was established.[13] Toward the end of the nineteenth century, in 1873, the first school of nursing in the United States was established at Bellevue Hospital in New York City. An independent institution modeled after Florence Nightingale's educational specifications, the Bellevue school was organized and administered by a board that had no ties to the hospital.[14] Public health did not exist as a profession until the early part of the twentieth century. Although public health courses had been an occasional part of the curriculum of medical, nursing, and dental schools, the first formalized school of public health was established in 1916 at the Johns Hopkins University through an appropriation from the Rockefeller Foundation.[15]

EXPANSION OF EDUCATIONAL PROGRAMS IN THE HEALTH FIELDS

Both the number and the kinds of instructional programs for occupations in the U.S. health care system have grown significantly since 1950. Although their increase can be attributed partly to the overall growth in higher education, it has largely resulted from the expansion of occupations within the health sciences and health care delivery and the need to develop corresponding educational programs. The broadening of health care delivery throughout the population, along with the rise of research in the health sciences, has led to a general increase in the number of personnel working in the health fields. Transformations in research and patient care, especially the use of the team approach, have in turn engendered many new occupations.

One hundred years ago, patient care consisted largely of the ministrations of individual practitioners of widely varying qualifications. The primary practitioners included physicians, nurses, midwives, apothecaries, and even ministers and veterinarians. In urban areas with many well-qualified practitioners, physicians led patient care activities, while other types of practitioner assumed secondary roles. In remote rural areas where trained physicians were scarce, however, midwives, nurses, apothecaries, and, in some instances, veterinarians frequently assumed the role of the primary health providers. Most of these practitioners made house calls and maintained offices in which they treated patients.

Today, by contrast, large teams of health care professionals are involved in treating individual patients, requiring the site of patient care to be moved from homes and practitioners' offices to hospitals and other health care delivery facilities. Another factor in this shift to treating patients in hospitals has been the ascending importance of the clinical laboratory in diagnosis and treatments. Physicians need, for example, x-rays and blood chemistry tests to properly diagnose and treat patients. A contemporary health care delivery team includes as many as twenty or thirty highly specialized workers from a variety of occupations. A physician specialist usually serves as the "captain" of the team, which consists of other physician specialists, nurses, technicians, therapists, and so on. New, specialized occupations in nursing, technical assistance, and ancillary care have evolved largely in conjunction with the expansion of diagnostic and therapeutic procedures, the enactment of new social and economic policies, and new approaches to the distribution of responsibility in patient care. Fundamental changes in health care practice have led to the creation of criteria and standards for many of these new occupations. Events such as wars, civil unrest, and national disasters have also contributed to changes in patient care. For example, new modes of triage and emergency health services have been developed in military interventions and rescue operations. In addition social and economic factors, such as nursing shortages, have helped bring about new health care occupations.

Scientific research in the health fields, like scientific research in general, has evolved from the work of lone investigators in solitary laboratory settings to large collaborative projects that are intra- and interinstitutional, interdisciplinary, national, and international in scope. A century ago leading scientists primarily worked alone or with a small staff in one laboratory. Today scientists in the vanguard serve as principal investigators of collaborative networks of research teams that span various institutions and include a broad cross section of occupations. These large-scale collaborative approaches have now become the norm for research in the health fields.[16]

The team approach to scientific research and patient care has special implications for higher education. In the past fifty years, the introduction of many new occupations in the health fields has had a major impact on post-secondary educational institutions in the United States. At the same time that existing postsecondary educational institutions have expanded instructional programs to accommodate changing occupations in the health fields, new types of specialized educational institutions have evolved. The number of vocational schools specializing in the health technologies and the number of community colleges with programs for ancillary health occupations have greatly increased.

The AMA, the American Dental Association, and several specialty societies have largely been responsible for initiating certificate and degree programs in the new allied health occupations at a variety of institutions. Professional organizations in the fields of radiology and pathology in particular have taken the lead in developing certificate programs for allied health personnel in their respective fields. Professional, undergraduate, and graduate schools have introduced many more specialized degree programs in the health fields at the bachelor's, master's and doctoral degree levels.

Early in the twentieth century, educational institutions specializing in the health fields also became more involved in research. In the post–World War II years, the federal government, largely through the National Institutes of Health, allocated vast and unprecedented amounts of funding for conducting research and training research personnel in the health fields. With the infusion of postwar funding came major new incentives for research at educational institutions and health care delivery facilities.

Institutions with instructional programs in the health fields expanded both physically and intellectually to accommodate these funding opportunities. Special components for research evolved at the departmental level in the basic and applied clinical sciences divisions. Eventually these institutions became centers for research in addition to being centers for education and patient care.

The factors that have been most responsible for altering the occupations in the health fields have also had the greatest influence on changing educational institutions and instructional programs in the health fields. Advances in science and technology, the rise of ancillary care, reliance on technology in both research and patient care, the introduction of third-party reimbursement for health services, heightened social and economic concerns, grant and contractual funding for research, and tighter regulatory controls are among the key factors that have transformed not only the occupations but also the instructional programs in the health fields. These factors have contributed to the increase in and the diversity of occupations and programs.

From the middle to the latter part of the twentieth century, development in instructional programs has been commensurate with major changes in the health care system. As the activities of health care have expanded in scope and become more highly specialized, instructional programs have had to keep in close step. Programs in ancillary and technological training have increased significantly over the past two decades. At the same time, graduate specialization in the health, social, biological, and life sciences has been on the rise. Within schools of nursing, dentistry, pharmacy, and public health, programs now range from the paraprofessional to the doctoral levels, and schools of medicine are establishing doctoral programs in some life and biological sciences fields. Many of these educational institutions have also added programs in health policy, finance, and administration. In the latter part of the twentieth century, legislation and governmental funding continue to have a significant impact on instructional programs in the health fields. The passage of the Medicare Act in 1965 opened the door for many new occupations, and the equal opportunity legislation of the past three decades has afforded many new educational opportunities to ethnic minorities, women, the economically underprivileged, and the physically challenged.

The complexities and costs of late twentieth-century health services have led to demands for more intensive quality and cost controls. As a result, several new disciplines have emerged in the following areas: health policy and planning, health economics, health services research, and health administration. These highly technical areas of specialization play an increasingly important role in the activities of organizing, financing, and regulating the health fields. Various programs in these disciplines have arisen at the master and doctoral levels in educational institutions including schools of public health, business schools, and schools and departments of public policy, economics, and administration.

The social sciences have also had a major impact upon the health professions. In the past fifty years, many new occupations that emanated from the social sciences have evolved in the health fields. Professional specialization has largely occurred in the following areas: health behavior, ethics, history of health care, social determinants of health, social analysis of health care, environmental health, environmental engineering, occupational health, international health, and health education. Archivists need to be aware of the importance of documenting these educational programs because these new disciplines are playing a strategic role in shaping the present and future directions of the health fields.[17]

Despite the concentrated institutionalization of education and training in the health occupations, individual instructional programs are still largely controlled by external forces—by professional, educational, and medical associations, legislative bodies, and governmental agencies. As in the earlier apprenticeship tradition, professional health associations function somewhat as the medieval guilds did in defining criteria and setting standards for skilled work and ethics of practice; they establish the criteria for each field's specialized educational requirements.[18] Legislative bodies and governmental agencies represent the public interest by defining the suitability of these programs and monitoring their compliance with educational standards and regulations.

Because the incorporation of instruction with patient care can in some instances raise the cost of care, many health care delivery facilities have resisted or severed affiliations with instructional programs and educational institutions. Health care reforms that emphasize cost containment may require that new sources of funding be found for the practical training of health care professionals.

CLASSIFICATION OF OCCUPATIONS IN THE U.S. HEALTH CARE SYSTEM

The U.S. Department of Labor has defined sixteen broad areas in which most health care occupations are clustered. (See Table 5–2.) Three basic types of occupation can be found in each of these categories:

1. *Service occupations* deal primarily with the delivery of technical and clinical services.

TABLE 5–2   Areas in which most of the health care occupations are clustered

---

Clinical laboratory services
Dentistry
Dietetics and nutrition
Education
Health information and communication
Health services administration
Medicine
Nursing
Pharmacy
Psychology
Science and engineering
Social work
Technical instrumentation
Therapeutic Services
Veterinary medicine
Vision care

Source: Data from U.S. Department of Labor, Employment and Training Administration; and U.S. Department of Health, Education, and Welfare, Health Resources Administration. *Health Careers Guidebook* (Washington, D.C.: U.S. Department of Labor, 1979)

2. *Educational and research occupations* deal primarily with pedagogical activities and scientific studies. In the health fields, education and research are inextricably bound together. Researchers frequently teach their area of specialization, and many educators also engage in some aspect of clinical or scientific research.
3. *Combined occupations* involve the delivery of services in addition to education and research and are represented mainly by faculty in academic health centers, who are frequently engaged in patient care as well as research and education.

According to classifications of the Department of Education, preparation for occupations in the U.S. health care system is concentrated primarily in two broad educational fields—the health professions and related sciences and the biological sciences/life sciences.[19] The health professions and related sciences encompass the highly specific training programs for service occupations as well as related research occupations. They include groups of instructional programs that prepare individuals to provide

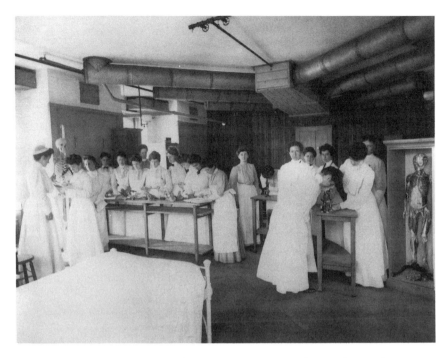

FIGURE 5–1   A class in gross and microscopic anatomy for nursing students, taught by Dr. Florence Sabin, the first woman to reach the rank of full professor in the Johns Hopkins University School of Medicine, circa 1915. *Source:* Alan Mason Chesney Medical Archives, Johns Hopkins Medical Institutions

patient care, or related research and support services, to individuals or groups.[20] The category of biological sciences/life sciences programs includes instructional programs that describe the scientific study of living organisms and their systems. Specialized programs in the biological and life sciences prepare students mainly for occupations in basic scientific research and education. Many of these basic science occupations are directly or indirectly part of the U.S. health care system. By providing basic instruction in the preclinical sciences, programs in the biological sciences also play an important role in the curriculum of specialized programs in the health sciences. Biological and life sciences programs prepare students primarily for occupations in laboratory research. (See Table 5–3 for a classification of fields in the health professions and related sciences, and Table 5–4 for a classification of fields in the life sciences and biological sciences.)

A dense network of controls and standards governs occupations in the health fields. Occupations involving patient care or research with human

TABLE 5–3 Classification of fields in the health professions and related sciences

Chiropractic
Communication disorders sciences
Community health services
Dentistry
Health and medical administrative services
Health and medical aides and assistants
Health and medical diagnostic and treatment services
Health and medical laboratory technologies/technicians
Health and medical preparatory programs
Medical basic sciences
Medical clinical services
Medicine
Mental health
Nursing
Optometry
Ophthalmic/optometric services
Osteopathic medicine
Pharmacy
Podiatry
Public health
Rehabilitation/therapeutic sciences
Veterinary medicine
Miscellaneous health sciences and allied health services (acupuncture and oriental medicine, medical dietetics, medical illustration, naturopathic medicine, psychoanalysis)

Source: Data from Robert L. Morgan, E. Stephen Hunt, and Judith M. Carpenter, *Classification of Instructional Programs* (Washington, D.C.: U.S. Department of Education, 1991)

subjects are the most tightly controlled and heavily regulated, from the education and training phase through credentialing and practice. Controls are exerted largely through the following four means: (1) establishment of criteria and standards for accrediting instructional programs, educational institutions, and health care delivery facilities; (2) licensure, (3) certification; and (4) regulations and legislation governing practice.

Accreditation is "the process by which an authorized agency or organi-

TABLE 5–4 Classification of fields in the life and biological sciences

Anatomy
Biochemistry
Biology
Biological immunology
Biometrics
Biophysics
Biostatistics
Biotechnology
Botany
Cell and molecular biology
Cytology
Ecology
Embryology
Epidemiology
Evolutionary biology
Genetics, plant and animal
Immunology
Marine/aquatic biology
Microbiology/bacteriology
Molecular biology
Mycology
Neuroscience
Nutritional sciences
Parasitology
Pharmacology
Physiology
Plant physiology
Psychology
Radiation biology/radiobiology
Toxicology
Virology
Zoology

Source: Data from Robert L. Morgan, E. Stephen Hunt, and Judith M. Carpenter, *Classification of Instructional Programs* (Washington, D.C.: U.S. Department of Education, 1990)

zation evaluates and recognizes a program of study or an institution as meeting certain predetermined qualifications or standards."[21] *Licensure* is "the process by which an agency of government grants permission to persons meeting predetermined qualifications to engage in a given occupation and/or to use a particular title; or, grants permission to institutions to perform specified functions within their jurisdiction."[22] *Certification* is "the process by which a nongovernmental agency or association grants recognition to an individual who has met certain predetermined qualifications specified by that agency or association."[23]

The most comprehensive sets of *legislation* governing health care practice are the Medical Practice Acts of the several states. This is "legislation valid within each state which defines and regulates the practice of medicine including qualifications for licensure within its jurisdiction." In some states the practice of physician's assistants, and other licensed health manpower is also regulated by the medical practice act.[24] In addition all states have legislation entitled Nurse Practice Act, governing the practice of nursing.

Another factor that affects instructional programs is the eligibility of the programs' graduates for third-party reimbursement and their ability to qualify in the competition for research grant funding. Service and research occupations that become ineligible for third-party reimbursement or fail to qualify to obtain grant funding usually have difficulty surviving. The pressure to meet professional standards for practice and to qualify for research funding or reimbursement of services are among the major economic forces that shape these instructional programs.

For the purpose of focusing this discussion, we have limited it to occupations with two or more of the following characteristics:

- Inclusion in the U.S. Department of Labor's categorization of occupations in the health fields (see Table 5–3);
- Existence of accredited instructional programs for the occupation;
- Recognition by legal, regulatory, and professional bodies of the right to practice the occupation;
- Eligibility of the occupation for either direct or indirect third-party reimbursement for services;
- Inclusion of the occupation on biomedical research teams; and
- Eligibility of the occupation for funding by research grants and contracts.

Occupations in the U.S. health care system are hierarchical and highly structured, ranging from the professional to the paraprofessional. The instructional programs for these occupations and the institutions in which the programs are based are equally diverse. In addition the range of credentials conferred by institutions with instructional programs is both extensive and varied.

THE ROLE OF ACCREDITATION IN DEFINING INSTRUCTIONAL PROGRAMS

In the United States, accreditation is a major process that links nearly all instructional programs in the health fields. Accreditation occurs at both the institutional and the program level. To be accredited, the institutions and the specialized programs at them must meet the exacting standards of official accrediting bodies. These bodies not only set criteria for accreditation but also confer accreditation status on institutions and programs. In the United States accreditation is voluntary in concept. Yet, because accreditation status is tied directly to the eligibility to receive governmental and private funds, the pursuit of accreditation has become imperative for the survival of institutions and programs. As a result, accreditation standards play a large role in the design and administration of instructional programs for occupations in the health fields.

Accreditation requirements account in large part for the standardization of instruction for specific occupations, which occurs primarily at the program level rather than at the institutional level. Basic requirements for specific degrees and training certificates are similar in all institutional settings. Because of accreditation standards, the curricula of specialized instructional programs tend to be both occupation- and discipline-specific. For instance, as a result of highly standardized nationwide requirements for nursing diploma programs, the types of core courses required for a diploma are essentially the same in every R.N. program.

The 1993 edition of the *Council of Postsecondary Accreditation Membership Directory* (the last edition before COPA voted itself out of existence) includes fifty-five associations. Twelve of the associations are responsible for institutional accreditation, the remaining forty-three are responsible for accrediting specialized programs at institutions of postsecondary education. Of the twelve associations that accredit institutions, ten are responsible for accrediting institutions that have programs for occupations in the health fields. (See Table 5–5.) Six of these associations for institutional accreditation are regional associations. Thirty-three of the forty-three associations that accredit specialized programs are devoted to programs for occupations in the U.S. health care system. (See Table 5–6.) The AMA's Committee on Allied Health Education and Accreditation serves as an umbrella agency for nineteen review committees, each representing

TABLE 5–5 Associations that accredit postsecondary educational institutions

---

National Associations

Accrediting Bureau of Health Education Schools

Career College Association
  Accrediting Commission for Independent Colleges and Schools;
  Accrediting Commission for Trade and Technical Schools

National Home Study Council

Accreditation Council for Continuing Medical Education

Regional Associations

Middle States Association of Colleges and Schools (Delaware, District of Columbia, Maryland, New Jersey, New York, Pennsylvania, Puerto Rico, Virgin Islands)

New England Association of Schools and Colleges (Connecticut, Maine, Massachusetts, New Hampshire, Rhode Island, Vermont)

North Central Association of Colleges and Schools (Arizona, Arkansas, Colorado, Illinois, Indiana, Iowa, Kansas, Michigan, Minnesota, Missouri, Nebraska, New Mexico, North Dakota, Ohio, Oklahoma, South Dakota, West Virginia, Wisconsin, Wyoming)

Northwest Association of Schools and Colleges (Alaska, Idaho, Montana, Nevada, Oregon, Utah, Washington)

Southern Association of Colleges and Schools (Alabama, Florida, Georgia, Kentucky, Louisiana, Mississippi, North Carolina, South Carolina, Tennessee, Texas, Virginia)

Western Association of Schools and Colleges (American Samoa, California, Guam, Hawaii, Trust Territory of the Pacific)

Source: Data from Council on Postsecondary Education, *COPA Membership Directory* (Washington, D.C.: COPA, 1992)

professional organizations collaborating in the accreditation of programs in designated allied health fields.[25] (See Table 5–7.) The principal accreditation group for schools of medicine is the Liason Committee on Medical Education, a joint committee of the AMA and the Association of American Medical Colleges. The Accreditation Council for Continuing Medical Education, an arm of the AMA, accredits institutions to approve continuing education credit hours.

Because programs for the health occupations are located in educational institutions and in health care delivery facilities, the accreditation of health care delivery facilities also plays an important role in the accreditation of instructional programs. The Joint Commission on Accreditation of Healthcare Organizations (JCAHO) also participates in the accreditation of

TABLE 5–6 Associations that accredit specialized programs in the health fields

Accrediting Bureau of Health Education Schools (medical assistant and medical laboratory technician)

Accrediting Commission on Education for Health Services Administration

American Association for Counseling and Development

American Council on Pharmaceutical Education

American Dental Association (dentistry and dental auxiliary programs)

American Dietetic Association

American Medical Association
    Committee on Allied Health Education and Accreditation
    Liaison Committee on Medical Education (with AAMC)

American Optometric Association

American Osteopathic Association

American Physical Therapy Association

American Podiatric Medical Association

American Psychological Association

American Speech-Language-Hearing Association

American Veterinary Medical Association

Association of American Medical Colleges
    Liaison Committee on Medical Education (with AMA)

Council on Accreditation of Nurse Anesthesia Educational Programs

Council on Chiropractic Education

Council on Education for Public Health

Council on Rehabilitation Education

Council on Social Work Education

National Accreditation Commission for Schools and Colleges of Acupuncture and Oriental Medicine

National Confederation of State Medical Examining and Licensing Boards

National League for Nursing
    Boards of Review for Baccalaureate and Higher Degree, Associate Degree, Diploma, and Practical Nursing Programs

---

The Committee on Allied Health Education and Accreditation (CAHEA) functions as an umbrella agency for nineteen review committees, each representing professional organizations collaborating in the accreditation of programs in designated allied health fields (see Table 5–7)

Source: Data from Council on Postsecondary Education, *COPA Membership Directory* (Washington, D.C.: COPA, 1992)

TABLE 5–7   Review committees under the AMA's Committee on Allied Health Education and Accreditation

---

Accreditation Review Committee on Education for the Anesthesiologist's Assistant

Committee on Accreditation of Specialist in Blood Bank Schools, American Association of Blood Banks

Joint Review Committee on Education in Cardiovascular Technology

Cytotechnology Programs Review Committee, American Society of Cytotechnology

Joint Review Committee on Education in Diagnostic Medical Sonography

Joint Review Committee on Education in Electroneurodiagnostic Technology

Joint Review Committee on Educational Programs for the EMT-Paramedic

National Accrediting Agency for Clinical Laboratory Sciences

Curriculum Review Board, American Association of Medical Assistants' Endowment

Accreditation Review Committee for the Medical Illustrator

Council on Education, American Health Information Management Association

Joint Review Committee on Educational Programs in Nuclear Medicine Technology

Accreditation Committee, American Physical Therapy Association

Joint Review Committee for Ophthalmic Medical Personnel, Joint Commission on Allied Health Personnel in Ophthalmology

Accreditation Committee for Perfusion Education

Accreditation Review Committee on Education for the Physician Assistant

Joint Review Committee on Education in Radiologic Technology

Joint Review Committee for Respiratory Therapy Education

Accreditation Review Committee on Education in Surgical Technology

---

Source: Data from Council on Postsecondary Education, *COPA Membership Directory* (Washington, D.C.: COPA, 1992)

instructional programs for occupations in the health fields. In addition, the JCAHO makes specific recommendations for educational programs in the following areas: child and adolescent health, diagnostic radiology services, dietetic services, emergency services, infection control, library services, medical records, medical staff, nursing services, pathology and medical laboratory services, services for patient and family, pharmaceutical services, physical rehabilitation services, radiation oncology services, respiratory care services, social work services, special care units, and surgical and anesthesia services.[26]

THE IMPACT OF THE REGULATORY ENVIRONMENT ON INSTRUCTIONAL PROGRAMS

Regulatory requirements play a major role in shaping curricula and defining programs. The regulatory activities that control programs and institutions in many instances interact with the regulatory activities that control the practice of occupations in the health fields. Knowledge of the regulatory environment is particularly important because regulatory requirements carry many stipulations regarding the generation, maintenance, and disposition of documentation.

LICENSURE

State licensing boards in the health fields are the authoritative bodies that grant permission to institutions to perform designated functions, and to individuals to practice specific occupations and assume particular titles. Each state has licensing boards in numerous health occupations. Licensure is intended as a means of quality control for practicing in the health occupations and operating health care deliver facilities. Meant to offer society a measure of protection from incompetent practitioners and inadequate health care delivery facilities, licensure governs the rights of individuals to practice and of institutions to operate.

To ensure that graduates have smooth entry into the work force, instructional programs for the health occupations adapt curricula to meet standards for licensing in their particular state. Whereas certificate programs tend to address only the specific licensing requirements of the state in which the program is located, degree programs usually aspire to meet the national norm in licensing standards, affording their graduates more professional mobility at the entry level. Most schools, however, have instructional programs that go far beyond the minimum licensing requirements, and rarely do students from accredited institutions fail license examinations. Because standards for licensure vary from one state licensing board to another, efforts are under way to introduce standardized licensing examinations for a number of occupations in the health fields. Greater standardization should help normalize curricula and create greater mobility for graduates.

Since 1915 the National Board of Medical Examiners has assumed a leadership role in providing testing services for licensing physicians. Its mission includes preparing and administering high-caliber qualifying examinations; cooperating with state examining boards, state boards, and other bodies involved in educating and evaluating personnel in the health fields; engaging in ongoing research to assess the quality of education in the health fields and to improve the precision of their assessment techniques; and providing educational outreach regarding their testing methodologies and procedures.

In recent years the National Board has engaged in cooperative projects with other health professionals. Major instances of collaboration have occurred with the National Commission on the Certification of Physician Assistants and the National Council of State Boards of Nursing.[27]

CERTIFICATION

Although licensure is required by law, certification is a voluntary process in the health fields. Specialty boards of professional organizations set standards and regulate the certification process. Even though it is voluntary in concept, board certification is a widespread requirement for employment in the health occupations. By also setting standards for the curricula and accreditation of instructional programs, specialty boards have significantly influenced both specialized education and practice in the health fields. Specialty boards determine length of training, scope, and content of courses. Board certification, which is especially important for advancement in academia, is also a significant factor in setting fee schedules and in the third-party reimbursement process.

TYPES OF INSTRUCTIONAL PROGRAM

Programs for occupations in the U.S. health care system exist either as freestanding institutions, as components of college or university systems, or as divisions within professional schools. Universities and colleges prepare students for many types of health care occupation through accredited graduate or undergraduate degree programs. Typical graduates of these programs are occupational therapists (who earn a bachelor's degree in occupational therapy), physical therapists (who earn a bachelor's or a master's degree in physical therapy), physician assistants (who earn a bachelor's or master's degree or a professional certificate), and pharmacists (who earn either a bachelor's or doctor of pharmacy degree, depending on the area of pharmacy in which they intend to practice). Professional schools in dentistry, medicine, and other fields require undergraduate education as a prerequisite to admission.[28]

A considerable number of instructional programs, such as those preparing physician assistants, physical therapy assistants, phlebotomists, dental hygienists, and nurses, are offered as associate degree programs at two-year community and junior colleges. Two-year community, junior, and technical colleges as well as some specialized institutions also offer degree and certificate programs for specialized clerical personnel and technicians. In addition, two-year community colleges offer degree programs that prepare individuals for further training in one of the health care occupations.

Specialized degree programs often exist within a professional school. For example, some schools of public health offer, in addition to a master's degree in public health, a master's degree in health administration, and many physician assistant training programs are located in medical schools or in schools of allied health. Some ancillary care workers, such as radiologic technologists, receive training in specialized short-term training schools and programs or at vocational technical institutions. These programs are either freestanding or based in a university, college, or hospital. Another type of specialized program is the continuing education program, now required by many health care professions as a condition of maintaining licensure. Continuing education is discussed in detail later in this chapter.

The records of institutions with instructional programs in the health fields contain vital data and information that are regularly used by the institutions, faculty, and students to meet evidential requirements for accreditation, licensing, and certification. Archivists responsible for maintaining the records of these institutions should give special consideration to the various evidential uses of these records. They should also consider the primary resource value of the vast range of records from these institutions that may be viable for ongoing studies in the health, life, biological, and social sciences in some areas of the humanities.

FUNCTIONS OF INSTITUTIONS THAT CONFER CREDENTIALS FOR OCCUPATIONS IN THE U.S. HEALTH CARE SYSTEM

The primary function of a health educational or training institution is to prepare individuals for occupations in the health care system. Closely related to the education function are the functions of research and patient care. At an academic health center, the three functions of education, biomedical research, and patient care are interdependent. Administration, including financial management, human resource management, information management, and facilities management, is also a function of educational institutions, just as it is a function of all institutions and organizations.

EDUCATION

Education for health care professionals may be divided into four levels: undergraduate education, graduate education, postgraduate education, and continuing education. Not every health care occupation requires all four levels. The focus of most instructional programs is to prepare their graduates to meet and maintain professional licensing requirements. At graduation, an institution confers credentials on students, but this credentialing alone does not enable an individual to practice. In nearly every occupation involving patient care, program graduates must also obtain a license or certificate before they are permitted to practice. Therefore, in preparing students to practice nursing, medicine, or dentistry, for example, an instructional program must impart high professional standards and include a curriculum that will enable students to qualify for licensing or certification.

Postgraduate education is required for practicing medicine and for specialized practice in the fields of dentistry, nursing, optometry, pharmacy, podiatry, and veterinary medicine. After graduation from medical school, physicians must complete an internship, lasting one or two years, in an accredited graduate medical education program. After the internship, physicians usually complete a residency in the specialty in which they intend to practice.

Most physicians who practice a specialty seek certification by a specialty board, although board certification is not required for specialized practice. Board certification helps to legitimize a specialist's practice by ensuring that the physician meets certain qualifications and has the credentials needed to obtain and maintain certification. Eighty-five percent of physicians specialize in one of twenty-three specialties.[29] Some newer areas of specialization include preventive medicine, family medicine, and community medicine. Dentists, nurses, optometrists, pharmacists, physician assistants, podiatrists, and veterinarians may also specialize. In most of the health care professions, licensing boards and state governments require additional education and practical training for specialized practice.

Many health care professions require continuing education as a condition of maintaining a license to practice. For example, in the medical profession, twenty-three states require continuing medical education (CME) credits for re-registration of a physician's license to practice medicine. Ten specialty boards require CME credits for recertification. Eight state medical societies and seven specialty societies require CME credits as a condition of membership.[30]

The role of the educational institution in continuing education is to host or coordinate continuing education courses and to confer the credits. The institution selects the speakers and determines the course content. The courses and programs are often underwritten by a commercial venture such as a drug company.

Continuing education is designed to broaden the knowledge and upgrade the skills of practitioners throughout the course of their careers. Because of ongoing and extensive change in the health fields, continuing education has evolved as a principal means of keeping graduates current with the latest developments in their professions. In some instances the accrual of continuing education credits is a requirement for maintaining licensure and certification. A number of states have introduced legislation that requires personnel in a range of occupations, including nursing and medicine, to earn a stipulated number of continuing education credits per year to maintain their licensing and certification to practice.

Overall, the quality of preparatory education in the health fields is still considerably higher than that of the emerging area of continuing education. More rigorous controls are in place for preparatory education than for continuing education because no single mechanism exists to monitor the quality of continuing education systems in the health fields. Evaluation of continuing education is done on a voluntary basis and credits are issued on verification of attendance. In recent years both federal agencies and professional associations have become more actively involved in setting standards for continuing education in an effort to improve its overall quality.

Although continuing education is still largely a voluntary process, it is rapidly expanding out of market demand. Even where legislation and regulatory requirements do not require continuing education, enrollment figures are high. Students voluntarily requesting evaluation of their course work is a particularly significant characteristic of continuing education programs offered by educational institutions.[31] The American College of Physicians self-assessment exam is an example of physicians' need and regard for self-evaluation. Personnel in the health occupations, especially those at academic health centers, appear to be highly motivated by the ongoing need to retool and to learn new skills and procedures. A clear consensus exists among personnel in the health fields regarding the need for relevant and high-caliber continuing education courses.

In recent years professional associations, legislative bodies, and government agencies have entered the debate over controls and standards for continuing education in the health fields, declaring that the relationship between commercial sponsorship and continuing education is not healthy. In 1990 the U.S. Senate's Committee on Labor and Human Resources held hearings on the role of pharmaceutical companies in continuing education. At about this time the AMA released guidelines on gifts to physicians from industry. These guidelines were readily adopted by the Pharmaceutical Manufacturers Association. In addition, the Accreditation Council for Continuing Medical Education and the Food and Drug Administration recently introduced guidelines designed to limit drug companies' control of the content of the continuing education courses that they fund.[32]

RESEARCH

Research plays an integral role at institutions of higher education. Federal research grants and contracts are a key source of funding for institutions of higher education, particularly those involved with the health care system. The need to obtain external support for research has changed the character of educational institutions in the health fields—particularly medical schools—over the past four decades. Entry into the competition for research funding has forced these institutions to expand administrative activities and set new institutional agendas.[33] Because tuition for professional degree programs in the health fields usually falls short of true costs, there is extensive cross subsidy of teaching from research funding and patient care revenues. Research funding is used to pay the salaries of faculty members, for the education of graduate students, and for equipment, among other things. It has created a new set of loyalties for faculty, who feel more obligated to their funding source (e.g., a governmental agency, foundation, or corporation) than to their institution.[34] As a result, confusion often exists at educational institutions over the ownership of research records. The granting agencies, principal investigators, and the institutions where the research activities are conducted share responsibility for the maintenance of these records. Because most grants are awarded to institutions and not to individuals, however, the institutions have ownership rights to any equipment purchased by grant funds and to the products of research. Furthermore, because the institutions usually have ownership rights over the physical research records and their intellectual content, they may determine the policies governing retention and use of these records. For instance, when principal investigators move to other institutions, they are usually required to deposit the original records at the institution where the research was conducted and take copies with them. In deciding which institutions and which research projects to fund, funding agencies play a critical role in the fate of these institutions. Although the awards are based on peer review, the decisions of these agencies greatly influence what research is done, where it is done, and who does it. Success or failure to obtain research funding may alter the direction of instructional programs and may cause individual departments to thrive or wither at an institution. At academic health centers in particular there is concern that the pre-eminence of the research function may skew the direction of education and patient care.[35]

In addition to conducting research, faculty at institutions of higher education with instructional programs in the health sciences train students for research occupations. A considerable amount of time, effort, and money is put into training researchers. Individuals planning a research career in the life and biological sciences usually seek a Ph.D. degree, which could be earned from a program based in a medical school, a health sciences school other than a medical school (e.g., a school of nursing or public health), or a university. Those planning a research career in the health sciences seek either a Ph.D or an M.D. degree. Some researchers hold combined M.D. and Ph.D degrees, including graduates of Medical Scientist Training Programs. Students who seek careers in public health and areas such as health policy and theory also earn graduate level degrees. (For a comprehensive discussion of research institutions and the research function, see Chapter 4.)

PATIENT CARE

Educational institutions with instructional programs for health care occupations are involved in patient care, usually through affiliation with a health care delivery facility. Most instructional programs include a practical component that involves the student interacting with patients in a supervised setting. The administrative relationship between an educational institution and a health care delivery facility determines the degree to which the educational institution is also a health care delivery facility. For example, in many academic health centers practicing physicians hold appointments on the hospital staff and are faculty of the school of medicine. The faculty's clinical professional activities provide revenue for the school and educational opportunities for students. Where the organizational relationship is very close, administrative distinctions between the educational institution and the health care delivery facility tend to blur. As a result, documentation of the activities of the faculty and student trainees may be generated in both the hospital and medical school.

INSTITUTIONAL ADMINISTRATION

Educational institutions and health care delivery facilities with instructional programs in the health fields have especially complex administrative responsibilities because education in the health fields is densely regulated. A significant portion of the budgets of these institutions is devoted to administrative overhead, including salaries and the costs of storage and management of evidential materials that must be retained for legal and regulatory requirements.[36]

In general, the chief sources of income for most institutions with degree and certificate programs in the health fields (public, private, or church-operated) include revenue from clinical services, research and teaching grants, tuition, gifts, and endowments. Public- and church-operated institutions receive operating appropriations from the bodies that own them, and they obtain funding though the usual sources of patient fees, grants, gifts, tuition, and endowments. Privately operated institutions compete in both the private and public sector for funding.

The extensive collaboration between educational institutions and health care delivery facilities in patient care, research, and teaching account for many complexities over the jurisdiction of documentation. Much of the collaboration is interdepartmental and also intra- and interinstitutional. Some collaborative activities are local and regional in nature, but many are national or international in scope. Support for these activities usually comes from a wide variety of funding sources.

The administration of institutions with educational programs in the health fields is largely decentralized yet strongly hierarchical, with a clear distribution of responsibility and authority. Usually these institutions have governing boards, a chief operating officer and central administrative staff, and departmental chiefs with administrative staffs. Because of the importance of effective regulatory compliance, the administrative structure of these institutions has been designed to distribute administrative responsibility to the appropriate location of activity. Whereas the institutions are legally responsible for the administration of grants, they place direct responsibility on the departments that receive the grants to administer them according to the appropriate requirements. In turn the departments place the burden of responsibility on the principal investigators to uphold the terms of their award. These institutions emphasize individual responsibility in research as well as in patient care and education.

At institutions with instructional programs in the health fields, the individual departments have considerable power and authority. Scientific departments generate funding through grants, patents, and technical licensing; clinical departments generate revenue from fees for services. As a result of their capacity to generate income, the clinical and scientific departments have significant leverage with the central administration of their institution.

THE ROLE OF ACADEMIC HEALTH CENTERS

Because of the need to integrate academic studies and research with practical training, specialized centers have evolved that combine institutions of higher education with health care delivery facilities. The academic health center is the venue where these two types of institution come together and where much of the education for the health professions occurs. The three functions of education, research, and health care delivery (i.e., patient care and health promotion) converge at academic health centers.

As defined by the Association of Academic Health Centers, an academic health center includes "a school of medicine (allopathic or osteopathic), a teaching hospital, and at least one additional health education program (structured as a school or college or functioning within other units of the center)." An academic health center operates either as a component of a university, as part of a state university system, or as a freestanding institution.[37] The governance structures of academic health centers vary greatly.

In one model, institutions are governed by a board and chief executive officer of the medical center to whom the hospital director, dean of the school of medicine and deans of the other schools report. (Duke, the University of Pennsylvania, and many state schools follow this model.) In a second model, the school of medicine is part of a university that contracts with several completely independent hospitals to provide teaching facilities in clinical settings. (Harvard, Tufts, and some of the newer state schools such as the medical schools at the University of South Carolina follow this model.)

The central educational component at an academic health center is the school of medicine. Almost all medical schools are part of academic health centers.[39] Other components of academic health centers are, most frequently, schools of dentistry and nursing. Schools of pharmacy, allied health professions (such as medical technology, occupational therapy, physical therapy, and physician assistants), public health, optometry, and veterinary medicine may also be part of an academic health center. As well, academic health centers may offer graduate programs in health-related scientific fields.[40]

In 1992 the Council of Teaching Hospitals recognized 123 academic medical centers in the United States, and the Association of Academic Health Centers (AAHC) counted 97 members. According to the 1992 *Academic Health Centers Directory*, approximately 60 percent of academic health centers are publicly owned and 40 percent are private institutions. All AAHC members are composed of one to seven schools or programs for educating health care professionals; more than 75 percent have three or more schools. Members own or are affiliated with between one and twenty-seven hospitals, with the majority (about 63 percent) linked to between two and five hospitals. The American Hospital Association's annual statistical summary for 1990 (the 1991–1992 edition) identified 1,238 teaching hospitals, representing 19 percent of all U.S. hospitals. Of these, about one third were government owned (18 percent state and local, 12 percent federal) and the remainder were privately owned (67 percent not-for-profit, 3 percent for-profit).

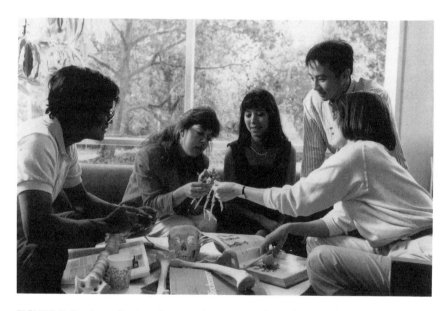

FIGURE 5–2   A medical student study group at the Johns Hopkins University School of Medicine, circa 1990. *Source:* Bill Dennison, photographer; the Alan Mason Chesney Medical Archives of the Johns Hopkins Medical Institutions

AN ACADEMIC HEALTH CENTER: THE JOHNS HOPKINS MEDICAL INSTITUTIONS

Like other academic health centers in the United States, the Johns Hopkins academic health center was initially organized around a consortium of professional schools, health care delivery facilities, and research institutes for the purpose of integrating the health care delivery (patient care and health promotion), education, and research functions. Recently, however, Johns Hopkins and a growing number of other academic health centers have opted to augment this consortium model to accommodate fundamental changes in financing and health care delivery. To stabilize the financial operations of its constituent institutions and to ensure their cost-effectiveness, Johns Hopkins added a vareity of companies that provide goods and services, including medical equipment, pharmaceuticals, and home health services, to its consortium. Many of these companies are also incorporated to serve the public sector. As a result the consortium includes a combination of for-profit and not-for-profit corporations, representing a notable departure from the predominantly non-profit consortium model for academic health centers.

At Johns Hopkins the consortium does not constitute a single legal entity. Unlike many academic health centers, the educational component (the Johns Hopkins University) does not own the consortium's health care delivery facilities. Thus, the educational component and the health care delivery facilities operate as separate corporate entities within a consortium that is dedicated to uniting the functions of education, patient care, and research at its constituent institutions.

The Johns Hopkins academic health center is currently organized around three corporate entities: the Johns Hopkins Health System Corporation, the Johns Hopkins Hospital, and the Johns Hopkins University. The Health System includes a network of smaller corporations that are either wholly-owned by the Health System Corporation or owned jointly with either the Johns Hopkins Hospital or the Johns Hopkins University. While most of these companies are not-for-profit corporations, several have been created as for-profit corporations. The purpose of the Johns Hopkins Health System is to provide an infrastructure of financial and service support for patient care, education, and research in the consortium.[41]

At Johns Hopkins the principal health care delivery facilities include the Johns Hopkins Hospital, the Francis Scott Key Medical Center, the Homewood Medical Center, and the Kennedy Krieger Institute. The health divisions of the university include the School of Hygiene and Public Health, the School of Medicine, the School of Nursing, and the Welch

Medical Library. The Johns Hopkins consortium of educational institutions, health care delivery facilities, and service corporations is one of the largest, most diverse, and most highly specialized academic health centers in the country.

The governance and administration of the Johns Hopkins academic health center is atypical in that there is no overarching governance structure and each of the corporate entities has its own chief executive officer and individual governance and administrative structure. Thus the Johns Hopkins Hospital, Health System, and University coexist as separate corporations with their own boards of trustees and chief executive officers. There is, however, cross-representation from the different corporations on the boards and within the administrative structure of the various organizations. For example, the president of the Hospital is also chief executive officer of the Health System; and the president of the University is chief executive officer of the health division of the University. Each of the professional schools in the health divisions is administered by a dean who reports to the president of the University. The director of the library reports to the dean of the School of Medicine who also serves as the vice president for the health divisions of the university. In addition, each of the university's health divisions has a faculty advisory board and each health care delivery facility has a medical staff advisory board.

OVERVIEW OF ARCHIVAL/RECORDS MANAGEMENT PROGRAMS AT ACADEMIC HEALTH CENTERS

The scarcity of published information about archival and records management programs at academic health centers led the Medical Archives of the Johns Hopkins Medical Institutions to conduct two surveys. In 1987 the staff sent questionnaires to 116 institutions designated as academic medical centers by the Council of Teaching Hospitals, and received completed questionnaires from 78. A majority of the respondents (53) reported that their institutions had repositories for historical records. In January 1988, the Medical Archives staff conducted a follow-up telephone survey of these 53 respondents. Although 40 institutions reported having archival programs, only 14 reported having records management programs. Interestingly, 13 institutions reported having both archival and records management programs, but in only four of these institutions were the two programs jointly administered. The survey results indicated that two of these joint programs were administered by university libraries, one by a history of medicine department, and one by the central administration of the medical center.[42] A majority of the archivists and records managers who were polled expressed alarm about the abundant production and accumulation of documentation at their academic medical centers. They were particularly concerned about the lack of archival and records management guidelines for the health fields. Many of them indicated the need for appraisal guidance that focuses on the special characteristics of documentation from the health fields. Determining what documentation should be selected and preserved seemed to be a priority in their work.

ISSUES IN DOCUMENTING INSTRUCTIONAL PROGRAMS IN THE HEALTH FIELDS

Degree programs in the health fields are generally based in institutions of higher education, and as such, their documentation falls under the purview of their institutional archives. While there is a need for appraisal guidance for documentation of these specific types of instructional programs, most colleges and universitites have an archival program in place.

Certificate and other non-degree programs, by contrast, are often ephemeral, as are many of the institutions that conduct them because they cannot appropriate sufficient funding. Those institutions that survive often lack archival programs. The archives of defunct specialized institutions are sometimes placed with the archives of their professional associations or accrediting bodies, which may themselves be deposited in large repositories. For example, records from various midwifery programs are located in the archives of the American College of Nurse-Midwives which are deposited in the National Library of Medicine.

A number of legal and regulatory requirements contain stipulations about the long-term retention of certain types of records from institutions in the U.S. health care system. In general provisions are made for retaining student records in both the degree and certificate programs. These records are regularly used throughout the careers of graduates. When graduates of these programs seek new licenses or admission to other educational programs, the application process nearly always requires that the degree- and certificate-granting institutions verify the graduates' academic credentials.

Granting agencies and philanthropic foundations are beginning to set more stringent requirements for the long-term retention of research documentation. In the meantime, insurance companies, professional associations, and federal and state agencies continue to impose many requirements for the long-term retention of clinical documentation. Because academic health centers in particular receive capital from many diverse yet highly regulated funding sources, they are obligated to follow varied requirements for the retention of fiscal documentation. As new data and information management technologies are introduced to institutions in the health fields, archivists at these institutions are challenged by numerous technical issues in the preservation and long-term use of institutional documentation.[43]

In summary, archivists at institutions with instructional programs in the health fields face many complex problems associated with the selection, organization, preservation, and ongoing use of documentation at their institutions. They need to be apprised of legal and regulatory requirements and well-informed about the ethical, social, economic, scientific, and technological issues associated with the institution's patient care, education, and research functions. These issues are indeed formidable, challenging archivists at these institutions to seek creative yet responsible solutions for the selection and long-term management of institutional documentation. Because of the need to plan carefully for the selection of documentation to be preserved, it is important for archivists to have an overview of the context of instructional programs at educational institutions and health care delivery facilities. By comparing their programs with others nationally, they will be able to identify the program's common and unique features which will help them to set priorities regarding the functions and activities selected for documentation. In concluding, our hope is that this chapter will provide useful background information for archivists as they develop documentation plans for institutions with instructional programs in the health fields.

ACKNOWLEDGMENTS

We are particularly grateful for the assistance of the following individuals from Johns Hopkins in the preparation of this chapter: Louise Cavagnaro—former vice president of the Johns Hopkins Hospital; Frances Dukissis, administrative secretary—Medical Archives; Elizabeth Fee, professor of health policy and managment—School of Hygiene and Public Health; Mary E. Foy, assistant dean and registrar—School of Medicine; Gloria Freeman, administrator for continuing education—School of Medicine; Carol J. Gray, dean—School of Nursing; Edward Morman, director of historical collections—Institute of the History of Medicine; Richard S. Ross, dean emeritus—School of Medicine; Patricia Stephens, director of scientific editing services—Welch Medical Library; and Arlowayne Swort, former associate dean for academic affairs—School of Nursing. We also extend special thanks to William G. Rothstein, professor of sociology—University of Maryland, Baltimore County, for reading earlier drafts of this chapter, and to Helen W. Samuels, head of special collections at the Massachusetts Institute of Technology, for sharing with us drafts of her work *Varsity Letters: Documenting Modern Colleges and Universities.*

NOTES

1. The functions that we ascribe to instructional programs in the health fields are corollaries to the functions that Helen Willa Samuels ascribes to institutions of higher education. In *Varsity Letters: Documenting Modern Colleges and Universities* (Metuchen, N.J.: Scarecrow Press, 1992), Samuels states that institutions of higher education embody the following seven functions: (1) confer credentials, (2) convey knowledge, (3) foster socialization, (4) conduct research, (5) sustain the institution (institutional administration), (6) provide public service, and (7) promote culture.
2. The U.S. Department of Education uses the term instructional programs to encompass educational and training programs.
3. In a personal communication with the authors, Arlowayne Swort (16 July 1993) noted that nursing programs have been especially costly to operate. She cites studies done in the 1970s and 1980s that showed that some hospital-based diploma nursing schools were more expensive than either associate or bachelor's degree programs. The cost imbalances between the hospital-based diploma programs and the nursing degree programs based in educational institutions led to the eventual closing of many hospital-based diploma programs. One probable explanation for the cost variables is institutional infrastructure. Because instruction for nursing as for other occupations in the health fields is labor intensive and heavily regulated, the cost of operating these programs is especially high. When clusters of these programs are based in educational institutions, many basic administrative and instructional costs may be shared. By contrast, the stand-alone diploma programs must assume the full brunt of administrative and instructional costs.
4. Council of Teaching Hospitals, Association of American Medical Colleges, *Committee Structure and Membership Directory 1991* (Washington, D.C.: Association of American Medical Colleges, 1991).
5. William G. Rothstein, letter to the authors, 24 Jan. 1993.
6. Ibid.
7. William G. Rothstein, *American Medical Schools and the Practice of Medicine: A History* (New York: Oxford University Press, 1987), 85–88.
8. Richard H. Shryock, *Medical Licensing in America, 1650–1965* (Baltimore: Johns Hopkins University Press, 1967).
9. William G. Rothstein, letter to the authors, 24 Jan. 1993.
10. James Bordley III and A. McGehee Harvey, *Two Centuries of American Medicine: 1776–1976* (Philadelphia: W. B. Saunders, 1976), 10.
11. Edward Kremers (revised by Glenn Sonnedecker), *Kremers and Urdang's History of Pharmacy* (Philadelphia: J. B. Lippincott, 1976), 227.

12. Ruth Roy Harris, *Dental Science in a New Age: A History of the National Institute of Dental Research* (Rockville, Md.: Montrose Press, 1989), 7–8.

13. Joseph Nathan Kane, *Famous First Facts: A Record of First Happenings, Discoveries, and Inventions in American History* (New York: H. W. Wilson, 1981), 687.

14. Rothstein, *American Medical Schools.*

15. Elizabeth Fee, *Disease and Discovery: A History of the Johns Hopkins School of Public Health, 1916–1939* (Baltimore: Johns Hopkins University Press, 1987).

16. See *AIP Study of Multi-Institutional Collaborations* (New York: Center for History of Physics/American Institute of Physics, 1992) for a report on the findings of this project, which aimed "to identify patterns of collaboration, define the scope of the documentation problems, field-test possible solutions, and recommend future actions to secure adequate documentation."

17. Elizabeth Fee, telephone conversation with the authors, October 1993.

18. For more information on professional associations, see Chapter 6.

19. Robert L. Morgan, E. Stephen Hunt, and Judith M. Carpenter, *Classification of Instructional Programs* (Washington, D.C.: U.S. Department of Education, 1991) contains a comprehensive list of the subfields of the health, life, and biological sciences.

20. Ibid., 169.

21. National Board of Medical Examiners, Committee on Goals and Priorities, *Evaluation in the Continuum of Medical Education: Report of the Committee on Goals and Priorities of the National Board of Medical Examiners,* (Philadelphia: National Board of Medical Examiners, 1973).

22. Ibid., 87.

23. Ibid., 85.

24. Ibid., 87.

25. Council on Postsecondary Education, *COPA Membership Directory* (Washington, D.C.: Council on Postsecondary Education, 1992).

26. *The Joint Commission 1990 Accreditation Manual for Hospitals* (Chicago: Joint Commission on Accreditation of Healthcare Organizations, 1989), 318.

27. National Board of Medical Examiners, *In Service to Medicine,* 75th anniversary publication (Philadelphia: National Board of Medical Examiners, 1990), 1, 68–70.

28. U.S. Department of Labor, *Occupational Outlook Handbook* (Washington, D.C.: U.S. Department of Labor, 1986).

29. Ibid.

30. American Medical Association, *1991 Continuing Medical Education Fact Sheet* (American Medical Association, Chicago, 1991).

31. Bordley and Harvey, *American Medicine,* 346.

32. Bonnie Davidson, "The New Ethical Climate of CME," *Physicians' Travel and Meeting Guide* (May 1992): 44–48.

33. Rothstein, *American Medical Schools,* 255.

34. Ibid., 248.

35. Jeremiah A. Barondess, "The Academic Health Center and the Public Agenda: Whose Three-Legged Stool?" *Annals of Internal Medicine* 115 (1991): 962–67.

36. David U. Himmelstein and Steffie Woolhandler, "Cost Without Benefit:

Administrative Waste in U.S. Health Care," *New England Journal of Medicine* 314, no.7 (19xx): 411–45.
37. Association of Academic Health Centers, *Directory* (Washington, D.C.: Association of Academic Health Centers, 1991).
38. Richard S. Ross, Letter to the authors, July 1993.
39. Rothstein, *American Medical Schools*, 225–26.
40. Joan D. Krizack, "Assessing the Context for Archival Programs in the Health Fields," in Nancy McCall and Lisa A. Mix, eds., *Designing Archival Programs to Advance Knowledge in the Health Fields.* (Baltimore: Johns Hopkins University Press, 1994).
41. The Johns Hopkins Health System includes the following corporations: Francis Scott Key Medical Center, the Johns Hopkins Medical Services Corporation, Broadway Medical Management Corporation, the Johns Hopkins Home Care Group, Dome Corporation, Broadway Services, Inc., Broadway Development Corporation, Johns Hopkins Pharmaquip, Inc., Johns Hopkins Home Health Services, Inc., Johns Hopkins Pediatrics-at-Home, Inc., Kennedy Krieger Institute, and Wyman Park Medical Associates, Inc.
42. Alan Mason Chesney Medical Archives, Johns Hopkins Medical Institutions, "Results of the Follow-up Survey of Archives and Records Management Programs at Academic Medical Centers" (unpublished). This survey was conducted as part of The Johns Hopkins Records Project, funded by the National Historical Publications and Records Commission.
43. See McCall and Mix, *Designing Archival Programs* for an in-depth study of how archives in the health field should function.

SELECT ANNOTATED BIBLIOGRAPHY
ACADEMIC HEALTH CENTERS

Association of Academic Health Centers. *Directory.* Washington, D.C.: Association of Academic Health Centers, 1991. Defines an academic health center; lists all members of the Association of Academic Health Centers, giving the members' component institutions and programs.

Barondess, Jeremiah A. "The Academic Health Center and the Public Agenda: Whose Three-Legged Stool?" *Annals of Internal Medicine* 115 (1991): 962–67. Discusses the relationship between education, research, and patient care at an academic health center.

Council of Teaching Hospitals, Association of American Medical Colleges. *Committee Structure and Membership Directory 1986.* Washington, D.C.: Association of American Medical Colleges, 1991. Lists all teaching hospitals in the United States, giving demographic information; defines the relationships between hospitals and schools of medicine.

Krizack, Joan D. "Assessing the Context for Archival Programs in the health fields." in *Designing Archival Programs in the Health Fields,* edited by Nancy

McCall and Lisa A. Mix. Baltimore: Johns Hopkins University Press, 1994. Uses the academic health center as a case study for a functional approach to documentation planning.

Munson, Fred C., and Thomas A. D'Aunno. *The University Hospital in the Academic Health Center: Finding the Right Relationship*, vol. 2. Washington, D.C.: Association of American Medical Colleges and Association of Academic Health Centers, 1987. Discusses the relationship between teaching hospitals and educational programs in the health fields.

ARCHIVES / DOCUMENTATION PLANNING

Samuels, Helen Willa. *Varsity Letters: Documenting Modern Colleges and Universities* Metuchen, N.J.: Scarecrow Press, 1992. Takes a functional approach to documenting educational institutions.

HEALTH OCCUPATIONS

Badasch, Shirley A., and Doreen S. Chesebro. *The Health Care Worker: An Introduction to Health Occupations,* 2nd ed. Englewood Cliffs, N.J.: Prentice-Hall, 1988. Provides background information about occupations in the health fields, giving educational requirements.

Morgan, Robert L., E. Stephen Hunt, and Judith M. Carpenter. *Classification of Instructional Programs,* 1990 ed. Washington, D.C.: U.S. Department of Education, 1991. Provides comprehensive lists of the components of educational programs in the health, life, and biological sciences.

U.S. Department of Labor, Bureau of Labor Statistics. *Occupational Outlook Handbook,* Bulletin 2250, 1986–87 ed. Washington, D.C.: U.S. Department of Labor, 1986. Provides Department of Labor designations for occupations in the health fields and descriptions of the educational requirements.

U.S. Department of Labor, Employment and Training Administration, U.S. Department of Health, Education, and Welfare, Health Resources Administration. *Health Careers Guidebook,* 4th ed. Washington, D.C.: U.S. Department of Labor, 1979. Lists all health occupations according to category; gives a detailed description of each occupation, including educational requirements, the nature of the work, and the state of the job market.

HISTORY OF THE HEALTH FIELDS / EDUCATION IN THE HEALTH FIELDS

Bordley, James, III, and A. McGehee Harvey. *Two Centuries of American Medicine: 1776–1976.* Philadelphia: W. B. Saunders, 1976. Covers the development of medical schools and education programs in the United States.

Fee, Elizabeth. *Disease and Discovery: A History of the Johns Hopkins School of Public Health.* Baltimore: Johns Hopkins University Press, 1987. A history of the first school of public health in the United States.

Harris, Ruth Roy. *Dental Science in a New Age: A History of the National Institute of Dental Research.* Rockville, Md.: Montrose Press, 1980. Discusses the history of dental education in the Unites States.

Kremers, Edward. *Kremers and Urdang's History of Pharmacy,* revised by Glenn Sonnedecker. Philadelphia: J. B. Lippincott, 1976. A comprehensive history of pharmacy in antiquity, the Middle Ages, Modern Europe and the United States; it includes a chapter on the development of American educational programs in the field of pharmacy.

Rothstein, William G. *American Medical Schools and the Practice of Medicine: A History.* New York: Oxford University Press, 1987. A thorough history of medical education in the Unites States, leading to a thoughtful analysis of the current situation.

REGULATION

Joint Commission on the Accreditation of Healthcare Organizations. *Accreditation Manual for Hospitals.* Chicago: Joint Commission on the Accreditation of Healthcare Organizations, 1989. Addresses accreditation requirements for hospitals. Issued annually.

National Board of Medical Examiners, Committee on Goals and Priorities. *Evaluation in the Continuum of Medical Education. Report of the Committee on Goals and Priorities of the National Board of Medical Examiners.* Philadelphia: National Board of Medical Examiners, 1973. A comprehensive discussion of accreditation, licensing, certification, and regulation in education for the health fields.

National Board of Medical Examiners. *In Service to Medicine,* 75th anniversary publication. Philadelphia: National Board of Medical Examiners, 1990. Provides historical information about licensing in the health professions.

Young, Kenneth E., Charles M. Chambers, H. R. Kells, et al. *Understanding Accreditation.* San Francisco: Jossey-Bass, 1983. A comprehensive discussion of the accreditation process; explains how accreditation came into being, what it entails today, the role of institutions, the role of accrediting bodies, and the relationship between accreditation and regulation.

CHAPTER 6

Professional and Voluntary Associations

JAMES G. CARSON

Professional and voluntary associations and organizations play a major role in the U.S. health care system. Professional associations serve as the collective voice of the various health professions, participate in and influence the regulation of those professions, and are a major force in educating and training health practitioners. Voluntary associations are significantly involved in providing information to the public on health matters as well as in funding biomedical research.

Gale's *Encyclopedia of Medical Organizations and Agencies*, the standard reference in this area, lists approximately 5,000 such organizations functioning at the international, national, and state levels.[1] Not included in this count are nearly 2,000 county medical societies[2] and untold local chapters of major national organizations such as the American Cancer Society and the American Heart Association.

Professional associations, as the term suggests, are organized around the concerns of particular health professions and draw their membership exclusively or primarily from practitioners of those professions. Their history in the United States dates to the founding of the first provincial medical society in New Jersey in 1766.[3] Such organizations act as the collective voice of the profession they represent. Their agendas commonly include enhancing the position of their own profession within the larger universe of health professions and in the eyes of governmental agencies and the public at large. Additionally, they devote themselves to setting requirements for licensure and maintaining standards for professional practice; to encouraging research, innovation, and education; and to legislative lobbying and similar "mutual protection" activities.[4] In terms of the functions of the U.S. health care system as presented in this work, professional associations are particularly active in two areas: education and policy formulation and regulation. Activities such as publishing journals and offering continuing education programs for members are examples of the educational function. Professional associations implement the policy formulation and regulation function through such activities as standard-setting and legislative lobbying. Some professional associations may also carry out activities in the realm of health promotion, and virtually all are involved to some extent in providing their members with practice-related products and services such as patient education brochures and job placement services. (This activity is to be distinguished from the U.S. health care system's function of providing goods and services, as defined in Chapter 1.)

Voluntary associations are typically organized around some particular disease, issue, or constituency other than a health profession. Examples are the American Cancer Society, the Planned Parenthood Federation of America, and New York City's Gay Men's Health Crisis. Depending on the nature of a voluntary association, its membership may consist predominantly of lay persons, or it may be a mixture of both lay persons and health professionals.

Voluntary health associations trace their beginnings in the United States at least as far back as the 1861 founding of the Civil War Sanitary Commission, devoted to promoting proper sanitation in Union Army troop quarters and to improving medical treatment for sick and wounded soldiers.[5] In peacetime, voluntary associations have made major contributions to the health of the American public by such means as promoting public acceptance of programs to control the spread of communicable diseases, initiating research projects, and sponsoring new health services unavailable through normal public health channels.[6] These purposes coincide neatly with three of the six major functions of the U.S. health care system: health promotion, biomedical research, and patient care.

In the latter part of the twentieth century, the health promotion function is the most prominent of the three in the agendas of these groups. The patient care activities of voluntary associations have largely been taken over by other entities. However, a few voluntary associations do participate directly in patient care—for example, by providing guide dogs for blind people, as do the Lions Clubs, or by rendering first aid to victims of disasters, as do Red Cross volunteers. A few other associations retain more indirect roles in patient care by funding institutions, such as the Shriners' burn institutes. The involvement of voluntary associations in the research function falls somewhere between these two extremes. Voluntary associations are rarely directly involved in carrying out biomedical research (with the notable exception of the American Red Cross); it is not unusual, however, for voluntary associations to fund laboratories at universities or other institutions.

Associations may occasionally move between the "voluntary" and "professional" poles over time, one example being the American Heart Association, which was originally organized as a professional society and later reorganized as a voluntary association.[7] In fact, the formation of associations is itself a typical aspect of professionalization. The medical historian Richard H. Shryock noted the deleterious impact of squabbles between practitioners on the *esprit de corps* of physicians in the early nineteenth century. Their responses to this state of affairs included agitating for improved medical education, promulgating and enforcing codes of professional ethics, and founding medical societies to place the collective weight of the profession behind these enterprises.[8] In a more modern example, the increasing professionalization of homeopathy is evident in the movement toward a uniform professional certification process for homeopathic practitioners and the consequent formation in late 1991 of the Council for Homeopathic Certification.[9]

The distinction between professional and voluntary organizations becomes somewhat fuzzy in areas of alternative medicine, which lack clear-cut credentialing procedures to define practitioners. For the most part, however, it remains useful to think of professional associations as those organized around the practice of specific health professions and of voluntary associations as those devoted to specific diseases, problems, issues, and constituencies in the health care universe.

The remainder of this chapter presents a typology of professional and voluntary health associations, with examples of each type. It then considers the functions of the health care system that involve associations and discusses the associations' activities that carry out those functions. Following these sections are two case studies: one of a professional association, the Illinois State Medical Society, and the other of a voluntary association, the American Heart Association. The concluding section gives a brief overview of current archival and records management activities among health associations.

TYPES OF PROFESSIONAL AND VOLUNTARY HEALTH ASSOCIATIONS

The universe of professional and voluntary health associations can be classified with reasonable accuracy into eight categories of concern or emphasis:

1. the medical profession in general;
2. medical specialties;
3. specific diseases or other medical conditions;
4. specific therapies or medical techniques;
5. allied professions and activities;
6. parallel professions;
7. alternative schools of medical practice; and
8. special concerns and constituencies.

As shown in Table 6–1, some of these categories contain both professional and voluntary associations, in the senses defined above; some include only one or the other.

In addition, one must note the existence of a class of umbrella organizations whose memberships consist of other organizations or institutions rather than of individuals. Some of these umbrella organizations fit relatively comfortably into one of the eight categories listed above. Examples include the Federation of Orthodontic Associations and the Federation of Prosthodontic Organizations, both of which include dental specialty associations; the Council of Medical Specialty Societies, whose constituency is clear from its title; and the National Health Council, whose

TABLE 6–1 Types of U.S. health associations, with examples

	Professional Association	Voluntary Association
General medical	American Medical Association	American Red Cross
Specialties	American College of Cardiology	—
Diseases	—	American Heart Association
Therapies/techniques	American Society of Transplant Surgeons	Living Bank
Allied professions	American Medical Writers Association	—
Parallel professions	American Dental Association	—
Alternative schools	American Holistic Medical Association	National Health Federation
Special concerns	National Medical Association	Gay Men's Health Crisis

constituency includes a variety of general health associations (both professional and voluntary). Other umbrella associations consist of institutions or organizations belonging to classes treated in other chapters of this work. The National Association of Medical Equipment Suppliers, for example, relates to the health industries; the American Hospital Association and the Council of Teaching Hospitals relate to health care delivery facilities; and the Association of American Medical Colleges, the National Association of Health Career Schools, and the American Association of Colleges of Nursing relate to educational institutions.

GENERAL MEDICAL PROFESSIONAL ASSOCIATIONS

The "arch-organization" under this rubric is the American Medical Association (AMA). Founded in 1847, the AMA exerted little influence during its first fifty years and only began to assume its current influential position after it was reorganized in 1901 into a confederation of state medical societies.[10] As currently constituted, the AMA is a professional guild whose membership of approximately 300,000 comprises slightly less than half of the M.D. physicians in the United States. (This proportion has declined slightly in recent years with the proliferation of medical specialties and the resulting competition for membership from specialty societies.)

Complementing the AMA are 54 state[11] and nearly 2,000 county medical societies whose membership consists of physicians practicing in a particular locality. The organization of the medical profession at this level considerably predates the formation of the AMA, and these societies are separate from the AMA. In a handful of states, however, membership in the AMA is a prerequisite to membership in the county and state societies.

GENERAL MEDICAL VOLUNTARY ASSOCIATIONS

Undoubtedly the most notable organization in this category is the American Red Cross, which has a professional staff of 23,000, nearly 2,800 local chapters, and 1.2 million trained volunteers. "The mission of the American Red Cross is to improve the quality of human life; to enhance self-reliance and concern for others; and to help people avoid, prepare for, and cope with emergencies."[12] In furthering this mission, the Red Cross engages in myriad activities, notably blood bank services and disaster relief—the latter an activity that typically involves patient care in the form of first aid. The Red Cross also has major commitments in the area of health promotion through such activities as blood pressure screening, first aid training, and AIDS information campaigns. Perhaps uniquely among voluntary health organizations, the Red Cross also operates its own biomedical research facility, the Jerome H. Holland Laboratory, concentrating on blood-related research.

MEDICAL SPECIALTIES—PROFESSIONAL ASSOCIATIONS

The professional associations in this category include about 80 specialty societies of physicians practicing medical specialties such as cardiology (American College of Cardiology), oncology (American Society of Clinical Oncology), family medicine (American Academy of Family Physicians), and the like.[13] These societies are similar in mission to the AMA, within the limits imposed by the particular specialties. They tend to compete for members with the AMA, which, as mentioned earlier, has lost membership (in percentage terms) as medical specialties have proliferated in number and complexity.

Alongside these societies exist numerous, generally smaller organizations devoted to subspecialties and interdisciplinary areas. Those related to oncology, for example, number approximately twenty, including the Society of Gynecologic Oncologists, the International Society for Preventive Oncology, and the International Association for Comparative Research on Leukemia and Related Diseases. Each major specialty features a similar constellation of subspecialty and interdisciplinary associations.

The Council of Medical Specialty Societies also deserves brief mention in this category. It is an umbrella organization founded in 1965 that now includes twenty-four member societies organized "to provide a forum and communications mechanism for the exchange of information . . . , to identify and discuss public and professional issues of mutual interest or concern, and to provide representation to appropriate organizations."[14]

Related to the specialty societies but distinct from them are the twenty-four certification boards organized under the American Board of Medical Specialties. These certifying boards, consisting of outstanding experienced practitioners, administer written and oral examinations in the various specialties and subspecialties. In 1993, 39 specialty and 72 subspecialty certificates were offered by these boards.[15] Although the members of a certifying board are likely to be members of appropriate specialty societies, there is no formal structural connection between the two.[16]

SPECIFIC DISEASES OR CONDITIONS—VOLUNTARY ASSOCIATIONS

This category includes such well-known organizations as the American Heart Association, the American Cancer Society, and the March of Dimes, as well as others devoted to a wide range of disorders such as alcoholism, Alzheimer's disease, and lupus erythematosus. These organizations typically include, in varying proportions, physicians, other health care professionals, and lay persons with a special interest in the disease or disorder in question. A number of the major ones (e.g., the American Cancer Society) are organized with state and local branches.[17] The American Heart Association also has a network of fourteen scientific councils consisting primarily of physicians practicing specialties related to its mission. These councils represent the respective specialties in the association's decisions on allocating grant support for research and in determining the content of the organization's professional education activities and public education programs.[18]

Also deserving brief mention under this heading are the Shriners,[19] a fraternal organization with a special interest in children's health and in burn research and treatment, and the 1.3 million–member Lions Clubs International, a service association that takes a particular interest in visually handicapped people[20] and funds goods and services such as eyeglasses, guide dogs, mobile glaucoma-screening clinics, and vision research.

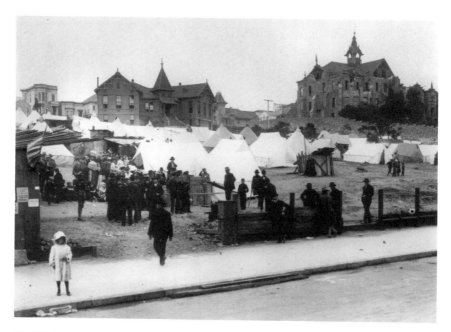

FIGURE 6–1   Shelters provided by the American Red Cross after the San Francisco earthquake in 1906. *Source:* American Red Cross, National Headquarters

SPECIFIC THERAPIES AND TECHNIQUES—PROFESSIONAL AND VOLUNTARY ASSOCIATIONS

Organizations devoted to individual therapies and techniques are organized around a large number of entirely mainstream health activities, such as organ transplantation and home health care; some less traditional but increasingly accepted techniques, such as biofeedback and acupuncture; and a handful of more controversial practices, such as cryonics (the freezing of a person's body after death, in anticipation of a future cure for the fatal disease) and Rolfing, a type of massage therapy. In the former cases, the distinction between professional and voluntary associations is generally clear. In the area of transplantation, for example, such professional associations as the Transplantation Society and the American Society of Transplant Surgeons are complemented by voluntary ones, preeminently the Living Bank and Medic Alert's Organ Donor program. To take an example from the opposite end of the spectrum, the Bay Area Cryonics Society consists of "individuals interested in life extension through cryonics."[21] In such a case—lacking a precise definition of what constitutes a "professional cryonicist"[22]—the distinction between professional and voluntary associations is difficult to draw with any degree of confidence.

ALLIED PROFESSIONS AND ACTIVITIES—PROFESSIONAL ASSOCIATIONS

Organizations devoted to professions such as nursing, medical records administration, and medical writing are included under this heading. The larger organizations, such as the 200,000-member American Nurses Association,[23] perform for their respective constituencies a range of functions similar to those of the AMA. Smaller organizations have less ambitious agendas, such as the American Medical Writers Association, which boasts 3,500 members and whose program consists largely of publications, an annual conference, and a thorough continuing education program.[24]

PARALLEL HEALTH PROFESSIONS—PROFESSIONAL ASSOCIATIONS

This category edges into the allied professions on the one hand and the "alternative schools" on the other hand. It clearly includes, however, a short list of professions: dentistry, optometry, pharmacy, and veterinary medicine. In general, these professions are characterized by the fact that their practitioners hold doctoral level academic degrees or have undergone a comparably rigorous pattern of professional training. Each of these has a national professional organization, such as the American Dental

Association and the American Optometric Association, similar in structure and function to the AMA. Both of these associations also have networks of associated state and, in the case of the American Dental Association, local organizations.

ALTERNATIVE SCHOOLS OF MEDICAL PRACTICE—PROFESSIONAL ASSOCIATIONS

Again, there is some fuzziness of boundaries distinguishing alternative schools from specialties or parallel professions. Nonetheless, some entities clearly fall into the first category; among them are homeopathy, holistic medicine, chiropractic, and naturopathy. Professional organizations in this realm include, for example, the American Holistic Medical Association, American Chiropractic Association, and American Association of Naturopathic Physicians.

ALTERNATIVE SCHOOLS OF MEDICAL PRACTICE—VOLUNTARY ASSOCIATIONS

Possibly the preeminent voluntary alternative medicine organization is the National Health Federation, the stated mission of which is to promote "individual freedom of choice in matters relating to health"[25]—which in practice means freedom to choose alternative as well as traditional therapeutic approaches. Some alternative medicine organizations seem to straddle the boundary between professional and voluntary. To take one example, the National Center for Homeopathy carries out both the educational function and the policy formulation and regulation function typical of professional associations, the former through its associated National Center for Instruction in Homeopathy and Homeotherapeutics,[26] the latter through the Council for Homeopathic Certification.[27] On the other hand, this organization also devotes itself to health promotion in a fashion typical of a voluntary association. For example, its annual meeting is open to the public, and it sponsors local study groups whose clientele consists largely of lay persons.[28]

SPECIAL CONCERNS—PROFESSIONAL ASSOCIATIONS

The preeminent examples of this category are professional associations for racial and ethnic minorities, such as the National Medical Association (NMA), the professional society of African-American physicians. Founded in 1895 and "[c]onceived in no spirit of racial exclusiveness, fostering no ethnic antagonism, but born of the exigencies of the American Environment, the National Medical Association has for its object the banding together for mutual cooperation and helpfulness the men and women of African descent who are legally and honorably engaged in the practice of medicine."[29] Although the need for such a parallel professional association has diminished somewhat in the ensuing years, the NMA continues as a forum for the special professional concerns of African-American physicians. Like the AMA, it publishes a journal and sponsors scientific meetings and continuing medical education courses, although it focuses on issues pertaining to economically disadvantaged and ethnic minority patients. Other examples of this class of associations are the National Black Nurses Association and groups of gay and lesbian physicians.

SPECIAL CONCERNS—VOLUNTARY ASSOCIATIONS

Organizations that include both health professionals and lay persons organized around a topic of special concern compose this category. One example is New York's Gay Men's Health Crisis, whose mission is "to provide support services to people with AIDS, people with AIDS-Related Complex (ARC) and the people who love and care for them; to [inform] the public at large, individuals at high risk for human immunodeficiency virus (HIV) infection, and health care professionals about AIDS; [and] to advocate for fair and effective AIDS public policy and funding."[30] Other similar groups include the Planned Parenthood Federation of America, whose mission encompasses public information and public policy advocacy related to contraception and reproductive health,[31] and the National Safety Council, whose mission is to "influence society to adopt safety and health policies, practices and procedures that prevent and mitigate human and economic losses arising from accidental causes and adverse occupational and environmental health exposures."[32]

TABLE 6–2 Role of health associations in the U.S. health care system

Association	Patient Care	Health Promotion	Biomedical Research
Professional	—	x	—
Voluntary	x	XXX	x

XXX, considerable involvement; x, minimal involvement; —, little or no involvement.

HEALTH CARE SYSTEM FUNCTIONS PERFORMED BY ASSOCIATIONS

As noted at the beginning of this chapter, professional and voluntary associations were once heavily involved in research and patient care. In the latter part of the twentieth century, however, three major functions of the U.S. health care system are significantly advanced by health associations: promoting health and health awareness on the part of the general public; educating and training health practitioners; and formulating policy for, and regulating the practice of, the health professions. In general, the professional associations are most concerned with the second and third of these functions, education and policy formulation and regulation, while health promotion looms larger on the agendas of the voluntary associations. A number of voluntary associations also carry out programs related to the research function (typically by funding research programs or institutions); a few also carry out patient care activities. (See Table 6-2 for a graphic representation of the role of health associations in the U.S. health care system.)

HEALTH PROMOTION FUNCTION—PROFESSIONAL ASSOCIATIONS

The health promotion function includes activities aimed at promoting health, such as fitness programs and informational campaigns. Though their principal focus is elsewhere, professional associations are by no means absent from this arena of activity. For example, the American Dental Association's stated mission includes promoting the dental health of the general public.[33] To that end, the association provides most of the dental health educational material used in the United States and sponsors the National Children's Dental Health Month program.[34] Similarly, the American Optometric Association sponsors an allied organization, the American

Education	Regulation/Policy Formation	Provision of Goods/ Services
XXX	XXX	—
x	—	—

Foundation for Vision Awareness, which supports public information campaigns focusing on the importance of comprehensive vision care.[35]

HEALTH PROMOTION FUNCTION—VOLUNTARY ASSOCIATIONS

The health promotion function is easily the most visible province of the voluntary associations. Often this function is carried out through public information campaigns. The National Safety Council, for example, produced media campaigns during 1991 focusing on water safety and the hazards of garage door openers.[36] The council also produces booklets and other publications for use in workplace safety training programs.[37] Health promotion may also be carried out in instructional programs for the public, such as the American Red Cross courses in first aid, cardiopulmonary resuscitation, and similar topics, which serve an annual total of 7 million people.[38]

Groups devoted to specific diseases also tend to focus largely on health promotion. The American Council on Alcoholism emphasizes public information activities to promote the prevention and early diagnosis of the disease and rehabilitation for its victims,[39] and the National Mental Health Association serves as the central national source for informational materials on mental health and mental illness.[40] The American Cancer Society's Cansurmount program trains volunteers with histories of cancer to provide functional and emotional support to cancer patients.[41]

Organizations devoted to non-mainstream therapeutic techniques and alternative schools of medical practice also tend to focus considerable effort on health promotion. Examples include the American Center for the Alexander Technique, which promotes a "technique that enables individuals to use their bodies with ease, grace, flexibility, and freedom from strain,"[42] and the National Center for Homeopathy, whose stated purpose is to "promote health through the use of homeopathic medicine."[43] In such cases, one may be inclined to question which is being promoted—the health of the public or the use of a particular technique or therapeutic approach. No doubt the organizations themselves would answer "both," as the above quotation from the National Center for Homeopathy suggests. However, even associations concerned with more mainstream therapies sometimes engage in promotional activities. A number of those concerned with transplantation, for example, have promotional programs designed to overcome public reluctance to donate organs.

EDUCATION FUNCTION—PROFESSIONAL ASSOCIATIONS

All the major types of professional association engage in educational activities, including general medical associations, specialty societies, and groups dedicated to specific treatments, allied professions, parallel professions, and alternative schools of medical practice. In general, the initial education for the health professions is delivered through academic institutions such as medical and nursing schools, with appropriate practical training in patient care settings such as teaching hospitals. Professional associations are not heavily involved in this aspect of the education function except that they typically participate in the regulation of educational programs by accreditation or similar processes. This is discussed later as an aspect of the policy formulation and regulation function.

Professional associations have also assumed a considerable role in activities designed to keep health practitioners abreast of developments in their fields. These activities include publications, meetings, and continuing professional education programs. Typically, health practitioners must participate regularly in formal continuing professional education as a requirement for retaining licensure to practice.

The AMA, for example, publishes the well-known *Journal of the American Medical Association*, and 10 specialty journals. The AMA also offers an ongoing program of continuing education for physicians at its Chicago headquarters, and offers practical advice to its members through its Practice Management Department. The American College of Cardiology considers that "continuing medical education is the College's principal priority" and operates a wide variety of continuing education programs. These include more than thirty programs on specialized topics offered annually at the college's Bethesda, Maryland, headquarters; a similar number of extramural programs offered at sites throughout the United States; and the annual Scientific Session, featuring over 1,000 reports of original research, lectures, and similar presentations.[44] The Association of Surgical Technologists places special emphasis on training practitioners to pass the national certifying examination in surgical technology.[45]

EDUCATION FUNCTION—VOLUNTARY ASSOCIATIONS

The education function is dominated by the professional associations, since participants in this function are generally health professionals. However, participation by voluntary organizations is not unknown. For example, the Eye Bank Association of America, a voluntary association focused on a particular therapy, operates a program to train technicians in enucleating (removing) eyes for transplant.[46] The Epilepsy Foundation of America supports professional as well as public education on epilepsy, principally by funding fellowships in the medical and behavioral sciences.[47] Organizations devoted to alternative schools of medical practice often are obliged to place great emphasis on education and training, since they may well be the only avenues through which such training is available. For example, the Himalayan International Institute of Yoga Science and Philosophy of the U.S.A. "operates . . . a graduate school, which offers masters degrees in Eastern Studies and Comparative Psychology."[48]

POLICY FORMULATION AND REGULATION FUNCTION—
PROFESSIONAL ASSOCIATIONS

Most professional associations perform activities related to the policy formulation and regulation function. Policy formulation involves coordinating health care services within a specified region or jurisdiction on a suprainstitutional level. In the nature of the case, activities aimed at implementing this function fall primarily to government and quasi-governmental agencies. However, associations do involve themselves indirectly in this area, typically through legislative lobbying to influence policy. The AMA, among its other activities, "represents the profession before Congress and governmental agencies."[49] In the specific realm of legislative lobbying, the AMA has in some years outspent all other organizations.[50] It has been joined in the lobbying trenches by other national organizations such as the American Dental Association, American Nurses Association, and American Hospital Association.[51]

Another type of policy activity in which professional associations engage is the consideration and formal adoption of policy statements on various issues by the membership, typically through resolutions of a legislative body such as the AMA's House of Delegates. Although this activity does not directly affect health care delivery policy as formulated and enforced by governmental and quasi-governmental agencies, it makes an association's views known and feeds them into the policy-making process.

Professional associations also engage in nonlegislative regulation activities, regulation being defined as the setting of standards for health practitioners and institutions. The most important and noteworthy instance of such activity is the participation of professional associations in accrediting education programs. The AMA, for example, cooperates with other entities to set standards for hospitals, residency programs, medical schools, and continuing medical education courses[52]; it also participates in the accreditation process for nearly twenty allied health fields. The American Dental Association inspects and accredits dental schools as well as schools for dental assistants, hygienists, and laboratory technicians.[53] The American Nurses Association issues published standards for the profession,[54] and the National Association for the Advancement of Psychoanalysis and the American Boards for Accreditation and Certification (one organization, its title notwithstanding) sets certification standards for individual psychoanalysts and psychoanalytic therapists.[55]

One conspicuous regulatory activity—the certification of individual medical specialists—is largely absent from the agendas of the professional associations, since it is generally performed by a separate system of specialty boards that have no formal connections with the specialty societies. Another such activity, discipline for infractions of professional standards, is usually carried out at the local level, by a state or county medical society rather than the AMA.

POLICY FORMULATION AND REGULATION FUNCTION—VOLUNTARY ASSOCIATIONS

As discussed earlier, policy formulation and regulation for health professions are carried out preeminently by professional associations in conjunction with other entities such as governmental agencies. Voluntary associations are not appreciably involved in many aspects of this function, such as certifying practitioners and regulating training programs. Other activities supporting this function are, however, sometimes found on the agendas of voluntary associations. For example, the American Council on Alcoholism lists, among its activities, supplying expert witnesses in state and federal proceedings involving alcohol issues.[56] The Epilepsy Foundation of America provides expert testimony in federal and state legislative proceedings and enters amicus briefs in court cases affecting individuals with epilepsy.[57]

A number of large voluntary associations are considerably active on the legislative lobbying front. For example, the cigarette-smoking ban on domestic airline flights is largely the result of a cooperative lobbying effort by the American Heart Association, the American Cancer Society, and the American Lung Association.[58] The National Safety Council has joined with the National Highway Traffic Safety Administration and the National Transportation Safety Board in an effort to encourage the adoption of state laws mandating suspension or revocation of driver's licenses of persons found driving under the influence of drugs or alcohol.[59]

OTHER FUNCTIONS OF PROFESSIONAL AND VOLUNTARY ASSOCIATIONS

As previously discussed, most of the functions of voluntary organizations fall into the health promotion and education realms. However, a few such associations are also involved in other health care system functions. These include, to a small extent, patient care, and to a larger extent biomedical research. A few voluntary associations do play a role in patient care by funding goods and services for persons suffering from particular conditions. One example is the mission of the Lions Clubs to aid visually handicapped people, which involves providing eyeglasses, guide dogs, and mobile glaucoma-screening clinics. Another example is found in New York's Gay Men's Health Crisis and similar organizations devoted to people with AIDS and HIV infection. The Gay Men's Health Crisis is heavily involved in providing direct patient services, though these services are for the most part complementary to medical treatment as such. Services include meals-on-wheels programs, assistance with shopping and household tasks, and legal and advocacy services.[60] A few other voluntary associations also participate indirectly in providing patient care by funding institutions, such as the Shriners' burn institutes. A more direct role in patient care is taken by the Planned Parenthood Federation, which has a network of over 900 health care delivery facilities.[61]

Research grant programs are funded by a number of groups such as the American Cancer Society and the American Heart Association. In other cases—notably, again, the Lions and the Shriners—voluntary associations sponsor research institutions focusing on their particular areas of interest. One exceptional voluntary association, the American Red Cross, operates its own biomedical research laboratory. The Jerome H. Holland Laboratory for the Biomedical Sciences, in Montgomery County, Maryland, opened in 1987.[62]

While many of the functions of professional organizations fall into the education, regulation and policy formulation areas, brief mention should be made of one additional distinctive function that is not a function of the U.S. health care system per se: the provision of various *membership services* to practitioners. Professional associations, including the American Dental Association and the AMA, have become major providers of professional liability and other types of insurance to their members. Many, if not most, facilitate professional placement by publishing notices of available vacancies and/or by operating formal placement services. Some also offer nonprofessional group services, such as mutual funds and other investment opportunities. Finally, virtually every professional association markets patient information brochures and similar materials to its members. This last activity may appear to straddle the functional boundaries between health promotion, patient care, and the provision of goods and services, but it is too prominent to neglect.

The advocacy activities of special-constituency groups also deserve brief notice in this category. To take an example, the National Black

Nurses Association espouses the role of advocate for improved health care in the African-American community.[63] Although such activities bear some resemblance to both education and health promotion, they are focused on the awareness of issues rather than directly on the preservation or restoration of health, and hence deserve to be considered as distinct from either of those functions.

Finally, both professional and voluntary associations must devote a portion of their attention and resources to the *administrative function*. Again, this is not a distinctive function of the U.S. health care system, but refers to those dealings with people, property, and money that any organization must carry on to survive. In general, these functions in health associations appear similar to their counterparts in other types of association. The organizational chart of the American College of Cardiology, for example, reveals a group of administrative committees with titles like "Budget, Finance and Investment," "Buildings, Grounds and Acquisitions," "Strategic Planning," and so forth.[64] Their counterparts in the American Heart Association's Chicago chapter include "Budget, Finance and Audit," "Management Services," and "Long Range Planning."[65] Both professional and voluntary associations also share such administrative activities as maintaining membership data bases, planning and executing conventions, and interviewing and hiring personnel. Many voluntary health associations also devote considerable resources to fund raising. For example, the American Heart Association describes "revenue generation" as one of its three principal enterprises.

FUNCTIONS OF UMBRELLA ORGANIZATIONS

The functions carried out by the umbrella associations naturally vary with their mission and constituency. In the main, however, they tend to cluster in the realms of education and policy formulation and regulation (which are also the two main areas of concern to the larger class of professional associations catering to individuals). Examples of the education function include management education programs for medical school deans and teaching hospital directors offered by the Association of American Medical Colleges,[66] the American Hospital Association's in-service education programs for hospital personnel,[67] and a series of executive development seminars for new and aspiring deans of nursing offered by the American Association of Colleges of Nursing.[68] Examples of the regulation and policy formulation function include the efforts of the National Health Council to secure uniform standards of financial reporting for voluntary health associations[69]; the National Association of Health Career Schools, which cooperates with governments and other organizations to maintain appropriate standards and policies in the realm of health career training[70]; and the National Association of Medical Equipment Suppliers, whose lobbying influence is hinted at by its stated interest in "support[ing] legislation and regulations that are beneficial to the home health care industry and provide incentives for suppliers to continue to serve Medicare/Medicaid beneficiaries."[71]

In some cases one function is overwhelmingly emphasized, owing to the special nature of an organization's mission. Such is the case, for example, with the Joint Commission on Accreditation of Healthcare Organizations (JCAHO), a policy-formulating and regulating body by its nature. JCAHO unites the American Dental Association, American College of Physicians, American College of Surgeons, American Hospital Association, AMA, and the public at large to establish standards and conduct accreditation programs for hospitals, mental health centers, hospice programs, and similar health care institutions and organizations.[72] The Association of American Medical Colleges demonstrates a similar overwhelming emphasis on the education function; alongside its many general activities in support of medical education, this association also administers the Medical College Admissions Test, a near-universal requirement for admission to medical school.[73]

CASE STUDIES

PROFESSIONAL ASSOCIATION CASE STUDY: ILLINOIS STATE MEDICAL SOCIETY

A typical medical professional society, the Illinois State Medical Society (ISMS) celebrated its sesquicentennial in 1990. Thus, its 1840 founding antedated by seven years the organization of the AMA. ISMS is now among the half-dozen or so "unified" state medical societies—that is, concurrent membership in the AMA is required of ISMS members. In 1990, ISMS had a membership of about 18,000, a staff of nearly 200, and an annual budget of approximately $6.4 million. The society states as its mission "to unite the [Illinois] medical profession behind: (1) promoting the science and art of medicine; (2) protecting public health; (3) elevating the standards of medical education; and (4) informing the public and the profession of the advancements in medical science and the advantages of proper medical care."[74] The education and health promotion functions emerge graphically from this mission statement; regulation and policy formulation are (as will shortly become apparent) implicit in the purpose of "promoting the science and art of medicine." (It should be noted that the ISMS mission statement uses "promoting" in the sense of "advancing" rather than the sense intended by the term "health promotion" as used in this work).

Health Promotion Function   Although it devotes most of its efforts to policy formulation and education, the ISMS noted in its 1990 annual report some health promotion activities, notably directed toward adolescents and senior citizens. The society's AIDS and Adolescents program, initiated in 1987, has sent more than 300 physicians into junior high and high schools across the state to teach students about the transmission and prevention of AIDS. The Partners for Health program, inaugurated in 1990, provides physician speakers to senior citizen facilities to make presentations aimed at improving communication between physicians and older patients.

Education Function   Education activities loom larger than any other single function in the reported 1990 programs of the ISMS. These activities included continuing professional education for practicing physicians—for example, producing and distributing an instructional video tape for physicians on HIV counseling and testing, and gathering and distributing information to physicians on contractual relationships with health maintenance organizations and preferred provider organizations. The ISMS also assisted in funding medical education by raising and contributing money to provide low-interest loans to medical students; and it engaged in education-related research, conducting a study of the merits of individualized continuing medical education programs.

Policy Formulation and Regulation Function   The 1990 annual report of the ISMS documented an active role for the organization in influencing health care legislation in the state of Illinois. In 1990 the ISMS was successful in securing passage of a bill providing immunity from civil lawsuits to physicians who volunteer time in community-based free medical clinics, and of another bill providing similar immunity to physicians who notify spouses of a patient's positive HIV test. Also on the ISMS legislative agenda were bills mandating Medicare assignment as a requirement for licensure of physicians, and providing for a "Canadian-style" universal health care system, both of which the society opposed. Through its Third Party Payment Processes Committee, the society worked with the Illinois Department of Public Aid to improve access to prenatal care for recipients of public aid; and its political action committee, IMPAC, for the first time endorsed a candidate (the eventual winner) in Illinois's 1990 gubernatorial race. Society members were also involved in revising state regulations affecting ambulatory surgical treatment centers and clinical

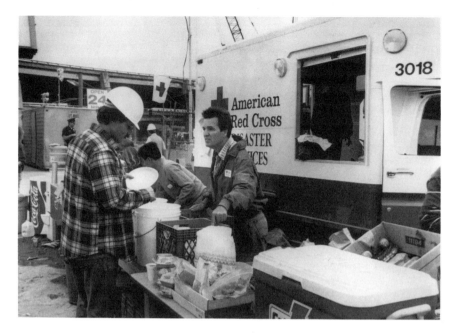

FIGURE 6–2   American Red Cross disaster relief services after the San Francisco earthquake in 1989. *Source:* American Red Cross, National Headquarters

laboratories, and the society was authorized to accredit continuing medical education sponsors in the state of Illinois.

Membership Services   Two noteworthy ancillary activities performed by the ISMS are examples of typical membership services. The society first considered the possibility of providing malpractice insurance in 1916, and its subsidiary organization, the Illinois State Medical Inter-Insurance Exchange, is now the seventh largest medical malpractice insurer in the United States. The society's biweekly newspaper, *Illinois Medicine,* while serving as a general news and educational vehicle for the profession, is also a principal advertising medium for job openings for physicians in Illinois and the surrounding area.

VOLUNTARY ASSOCIATION CASE STUDY: AMERICAN HEART ASSOCIATION

The American Heart Association (AHA) traces its beginnings to the founding of the Association for the Prevention and Relief of Heart Disease in New York City in 1915. This and similar groups in several other cities banded together to form the American Heart Association in 1924. At first the association consisted primarily of physicians and other health professionals. By the late 1930s, the membership had become increasingly interested in expanding its activities to reach the general public. Its first grant funding for a public information program, on rheumatic fever, was received from the American Legion in 1946. With this encouragement, the association was reorganized as a voluntary association in 1948.[75] From that time it began to involve lay persons with skills in fund raising, public information, business management, communications, and community organization.[76]

The AHA's simple, straightforward mission statement is as follows: "The mission of the American Heart Association is to reduce disability and death from cardiovascular diseases and stroke." The AHA carries on three principal activities in support of this mission: "cardiovascular research, cardiovascular education, and revenue generation." In terms of the division of functions used in this study, cardiovascular research corresponds to the research function, and cardiovascular education embraces both the education and the health promotion functions. The third activity, revenue generation, represents the enormous nationwide effort conducted by the association to raise funds for its other activities, largely through volunteer solicitation of gifts from individuals. As of 1992, the association included approximately 2,000 state and metropolitan affiliates, divisions, and branches, and involved some 3.5 million volunteers.

A unique feature of the AHA organization, the fourteen councils have a collective total of 18,200 members, primarily physicians and other health professionals. Each council is devoted to a particular specialized area. A few examples include councils on Cardiopulmonary and Critical Care, Cardiovascular Nursing, and Epidemiology and Prevention. The councils are represented on the AHA Research Committee, which oversees the allocation of research grants; the councils also give guidance to the AHA's professional education and public information initiatives.

Health Promotion Function   Given the general predominance of this function in the programs of most voluntary associations, it is not surprising to find that the AHA supports a wide array of community programs to reduce death and disability from heart and blood vessel diseases. These programs focus on a variety of topics, including heart attack, high blood pressure, rheumatic fever, stroke, congenital heart disease, nutrition, smoking, and cardiopulmonary resuscitation. Specific examples include Heart at Work, a program based in the workplace that was started in 1985 and focuses on risk factors and early warning signs of heart attack; an extensive arsenal of informational packages for elementary and high school audiences; and the Tobacco Free America Project, a cooperative enterprise with the American Cancer Society and American Lung Association. These programs collectively accounted for an expenditure of $55.9 million during the 1990–1991 fiscal year and reached nearly 25 million people. During the same period, AHA-sponsored cholesterol screening and blood pressure checks reached 1.3 million people.

The AHA also dispenses information to the public through print and electronic media; over 3,700 inquiries from members of the media were answered by the association's National Center during 1990–1991, while thousands more were handled by local affiliates.

Education Function   Perhaps reflecting its origins as a professional society, the AHA continues to be invested in professional education to a degree unusual for a voluntary association. Its 1990–1991 budget for this purpose was $30 million. The annual AHA Scientific Sessions, begun in 1925, are "now one of the nation's largest gathering[s] of scientists, physicians and other health professionals concerned about . . . cardiovascular diseases."[77] The association also publishes eight professional journals, including *Arteriosclerosis and Thrombosis: A Journal of Vascular Biology, Currents in Emergency Cardiac Care,* and *Heart Disease and Stroke,* a journal inaugurated in 1992 and targeted specifically at primary care physicians.

Policy Formulation and Regulation Function   As noted earlier, the involvement of voluntary associations in this function is somewhat limited, in comparison to the professional associations. The AHA is, however, among those voluntary associations with active lobbying presences in Washington, D.C. The AHA Office of Public Affairs was established in 1981 "to interact with Congress and federal regulatory agencies on such issues as biomedical research funding, tobacco control and nutrition."[78]

Other Functions   Not atypically for a major voluntary health association, the AHA's indirect involvement in biomedical research is considerable. In fact, the association provides more financial support for cardiovascular research than any other nongovernmental body in the world, primarily through fellowships for scientific investigators and grants-in-aid for specific projects. The association made a major commitment to increased research funding in the late 1980s, at least partly in response to the decline in federal support for such research. The first three AHA–Bugher Foundation Centers for Molecular Biology of the Cardiovascular System were opened in 1986, with the support of the Henrietta B. and Frederick H. Bugher Foundation, at Baylor University College of Medicine, in Houston, Texas, the University of Texas Southwestern Medical

Center, in Dallas; and Children's Hospital, in Boston. Three additional centers (at Brigham and Women's Hospital, in Boston, Stanford University, and the University of California at San Diego) were added in 1991.

"Revenue generation," of course, is hardly a function unique to the U.S health care system. However, since the AHA (with refreshing frankness) identifies this as one of its major enterprises, it might be noted in passing that the 1990–1991 income of the AHA reached $288.5 million. Of this total, $235.7 million was received as contributions from the general public. The AHA has also had significant success in attracting research funding from pharmaceutical companies and philanthropic foundations.

CURRENT ARCHIVAL/RECORDS MANAGEMENT PROGRAMS IN HEALTH ASSOCIATIONS

Not surprisingly, archival coverage of professional and voluntary health associations is spotty at best. Of approximately 2,800 individuals listed in the most recent (1991) membership directory of the Society of American Archivists, fifteen, or slightly more than one half of 1 percent, were employed by health associations. In all but one case, the employing associations were professional organizations such as the AMA and the American Hospital Association.[79] Of the roughly forty associations mentioned at one point or another in this chapter, eight are definitely known to have ongoing archival or records management programs. These include the American Hospital Association, AMA, American Dental Association, American Heart Association, American Optometric Association, Illinois State Medical Society, American Red Cross, and Planned Parenthood Federation. Most of these programs are operated on-site by personnel of the respective associations. In two cases, however, the association records are instead placed in external repositories: the records of the American Red Cross are transferred to the National Archives of the United States, and the records of the Planned Parenthood Federation are deposited in the Sophia Smith Collection at Smith College, in Northampton, Massachusetts.[80]

Several additional organizations—the American College of Cardiology, the Transplantation Society, and Lions Clubs International—have accumulated collections of historical materials, but it is not certain that these collections are managed, organized, or added to in any systematic fashion. Two additional associations, the American Academy of Family Physicians and the American Academy of Pediatrics, were in the process of beginning an archival program as of spring 1992. Thus, among the forty or so associations mentioned in this chapter, no more than one in four appears to maintain any sort of archival or records management program. If applied to the entire universe of perhaps 5,000 U.S. health associations, this ratio is in all likelihood misleadingly optimistic, given the fact that large and well-known associations are disproportionately represented among those treated in this chapter.

Some of the programs just mentioned, notably those of the American Dental Association, the American Optometric Association, and the American Hospital Association, are devoted to documenting the history of the respective professions as well as of the associations themselves. Several additional medical specialty societies identify themselves as maintaining discipline history centers for their respective specialties. These include the American Society of Anesthesiologists, American College of Physicians (for internal medicine), American Association of Neurological Surgeons, American College of Obstetrics and Gynecology, Oncology Nursing Society, American Academy of Ophthalmology, American Academy of Otolaryngology, and American Psychiatric Association. It is not clear, however, that the discipline history activities of these societies are always associated with an ongoing archival program comparable in scope to those of, for example, the American Dental Association or the American Hospital Association.

An example of a professional association archives is the American Medical Association Archives, located in the AMA headquarters building in Chicago, where it is staffed by one full-time employee[81] and holds approximately 3,000 cubic feet of material. The AMA Archives systematically preserves record copies of association publications as well as the official actions of the AMA House of Delegates and subsidiary committees and councils. The archives' holdings also include audiovisual materials prepared for public information purposes. However, it makes no consistent effort to collect unpublished material that would document the association's activities in the policy formulation and regulation realm, or in other areas that do not inherently involve the dispensing of information.

Among archival or records management programs in voluntary associations, that of the American Heart Association appears to be one of the best organized. The AHA employs one full-time records manager, supported by a budget of $3,850.[82] The program includes a written job description for the records manager and a multipage manual for the records management function that lists objectives for the program, characteristics of records to be targeted for preservation, and a sampling of types of record to be preserved. The reported holdings are approximately 50,000 documents, including annual reports, AHA journals and newsletters, by-laws, biographical materials, and numerous other types of documents.

These two examples are, as suggested above, highly atypical. Many other health associations are small, shoestring operations, and it should hardly be surprising to find that they lack the resources to place a high priority on the systematic documentation of their operations. Others—notably AIDS organizations—are growing explosively to meet expanding need, but may well prefer to devote all their resources to their primary missions rather than to documentation efforts.[83] This interpretation seems to be supported by one response to my request for information, that of the Gay Men's Health Crisis, which sent an impressive total of twenty-six pieces of AIDS information literature[84] while passing over the issue of archival/records management activities in complete silence.[85]

A related area of concern is the collecting of health association records by repositories outside the associations themselves. This topic was touched on briefly earlier in this section, with reference to the records of the American Red Cross and the Planned Parenthood Federation, which are deposited, respectively, in the National Archives of the United States and the Sophia Smith Collection at Smith College. In these two cases, the presence of the associations' records in the archives is the result of an ongoing cooperative arrangement between association and repository.

In many other cases, however, health association records are collected not under such continuing arrangements, but as a result of one-time transfers to external repositories. A search of standard national bibliographic resources for archival and manuscript collections revealed about 130 entries for health association records in external repositories—at first blush, a mildly encouraging figure.[86] However, the overwhelming majority of these entries—95 of 130—represent collections from state and local medical and specialty societies, deposited for the most part in university libraries or local historical societies.[87] Of the remaining thirty-five entries, about twenty represent state and local voluntary association records, from, for example, local Red Cross Chapters and the Wisconsin Lung Association, also preponderantly in university and historical society collections. Only about 15 entries represent national associations—ten professional (e.g., the American Society for Clinical Investigation and the American Association for Medical Systems and Informatics) and five voluntary (e.g., the American Council on Alcohol Problems, the Association for Voluntary Sterilization). Thus, at the national level, the collecting of archival and manuscript material from health associations seems to be, if anything, less commonplace among external repositories than among the associations themselves.

It seems clear, then, that in the realm of health associations there is need both for vastly increased documentation efforts and for shrewd priority-setting in those efforts, which obviously must be selective in terms of both organizations and functions targeted for documentation. It is hoped that this chapter provides a framework for making these difficult decisions.

ACKNOWLEDGMENTS

My first debt of gratitude is owed to Victoria A. Davis, who encouraged me to continue her work on this project after her departure from the American Medical Association. I wish to thank the staffs of the AMA library and the library systems of the University of Illinois at Chicago and Loyola University of Chicago. For assistance in gaining access to these libraries, I thank the late Ann Faulkner, formerly Assistant Dean of the Graduate School at Loyola, and Karen Graves, formerly at the AMA, now acting documents librarian at the University of Illinois at Chicago.

I also thank association staff members who went to considerable trouble to provide me with information about their respective associations: Rebecca Rhine Gschwend, Council of Medical Specialty Societies; Susan Lucius, American Heart Association (National Center); Lynn Gigliotti, American Heart Association of Metropolitan Chicago; Linda Hudson, Illinois State Medical Society; Jerry Knoll, American Red Cross; Charlotte A. Rancilio, American Optometric Association; Jennifer C. Wellman, National Center for Homeopathy; Patrick F. Cannon, Lions Clubs International; Robert W. O'Brien, National Safety Council; Suzanne H. Howard, American College of Cardiology; Patrick Giles, Gay Men's Health Crisis; Gloria A. Roberts, Planned Parenthood Federation of America; Michelle Armstrong, Association of Surgical Technologists; and J. Lee Dockerly, American Board of Medical Specialties. I am also grateful to archival consultant Cynthia Swank, of the Inlook Group, for information on the Epilepsy Foundation of America, and to fellow author Peter Hirtle, of the National Archives and Records Administration, for assistance with online searching of the Research Libraries Information Network.

NOTES

1. *Encyclopedia of Medical Organizations and Agencies* (Detroit: Gale Research, 1987 [2nd ed.], 1990 [3rd ed.], and 1992 [4th ed.]) (hereafter cited as *EMOA-2, EMOA-3,* and *EMOA-4,* respectively). The actual number of listings in *EMOA* is over 12,000; however, this count includes government agencies, funding

organizations, and research centers and institutes, all of which fall outside the scope of this chapter.

2. Paul J. Feldstein, *Health Associations and the Demand for Legislation: The Political Economy of Health* (Cambridge, Mass.: Ballinger, 1977), 28.

3. Paul Starr, *The Social Transformation of American Medicine: The Rise of a Sovereign Profession and the Making of a Vast Industry* (New York: Basic Books, 1982), 40.

4. James M. Rosser and Howard E. Mossberg, *An Analysis of Health Care Delivery* (New York: John Wiley & Sons, 1977), 33–34.

5. Page Smith, *Trial by Fire: A People's History of the Civil War and Reconstruction* (New York: McGraw-Hill, 1982), 393–99.

6. Lloyd E. Burton and Hugh H. Smith, *Public Health and Community Medicine* (Baltimore: Williams & Wilkins, 1970) 60. Quoted in Rosser and Mossberg, *Health Care Delivery*, 29.

7. These events took place in 1924 and 1948, respectively. The American Heart Association is discussed as a case study in a later section of this chapter.

8. Richard H. Shryock, *The Development of Modern Medicine* (Madison: University of Wisconsin Press, 1979), 267, and *Medicine in America: Historical Essays* (Baltimore: Johns Hopkins Press, 1966), 154, 157.

9. *Homeopathy Today*, April 1992 (Fairfax, Va.: National Center for Homeopathy), 21.

10. Starr, *American Medicine*, 91, 109. In 1901 the AMA House of Delegates was established, with membership drawn primarily from representatives of the state societies in proportion to the states' membership. This replaced the previous haphazard system that gave undue influence to physicians who lived near the sites of annual meetings. The change provided greater continuity and authority in the AMA's own decision-making and gave rise to dramatic increases in the state societies' membership and influence.

11. The count of 54 includes the 50 states plus "state-type" associations in the District of Columbia, Guam, Puerto Rico, and the Virgin Islands.

12. "The American Red Cross: People Helping People" (American National Red Cross, Washington, D.C.: 1989, Brochure). This information about the Red Cross is drawn from recent publications provided by the organization itself.

13. Since medical specialties are, by definition, health professions, there are no voluntary associations devoted to medical specialties as such.

14. Council of Medical Specialty Societies Mission Statement (Council of Medical Specialty Societies, Lake Forest, Ill. February 1992).

15. J. Lee Dockery, M.D., Executive Vice President, American Board of Medical Specialties, telephone conversation with author, 2 Nov. 1993. The actual number of distinct subspecialties in which certificates are offered is somewhat less than 72 because of overlap among the subspecialty certificates offered by the 24 boards; for example, the boards in family practice, internal medicine, and pediatrics all offer subspecialty certification in sports medicine.

16. Rebecca Rhine Gschwend, Acting Executive Vice President, Council of Medical Specialty Societies, telephone conversation with author, 18 May 1992. Informal relationships between specialty certification boards and

specialty societies reportedly run the gamut from close cooperation to mutual suspicion and antagonism.

17. This is both similar to and in contrast with the relationship between the AMA and the state and local medical societies, which are separate but related organizations, rather than "chapters" or "branches" of the AMA.

18. American Heart Association, *American Heart Association Scientific Councils and Journals* (Dallas: American Heart Association, 1991), 1.

19. The full name of the Shriners is the Imperial Council of the Ancient Arabic Order of the Nobles of the Mystic Shrine for North America.

20. *EMOA-2*, 758.

21. *EMOA-2*, 235. This organization is not listed in the third or fourth editions.

22. The Bay Area Cryonics Society did not respond to my request for a statement of its views on this issue of definition.

23. *EMOA-4*, 644.

24. This information is drawn from recent brochures provided by the association.

25. *EMOA-4*, 23.

26. Advertisement for 70th annual summer instructional program, *Homeopathy Today*, April 1992, 18.

27. Harry F. Swope, and Randall Neustaedter, "Council for Homeopathic Certification moves ahead," *Homeopathy Today*, April 1992, 21.

28. National Center for Homeopathy, *Homeopathy: Natural Medicine for the 21st Century* (Fairfax, Va.: National Center for Homeopathy, 1992), 7–8.

29. This statement, written in 1908 by Charles V. Roman, a past president of the NMA, is carried on the title page of every issue of the NMA *Journal.*

30. "GMHC: First in the Fight Against AIDS" (Gay Men's Health Crisis, New York, 1992, Brochure).

31. "Mission and Policy Statements" (Planned Parenthood Federation of America, New York, 1990), 2.

32. National Safety Council, *Looking Toward Tomorrow: 1991 Report to the Nation* (Chicago: National Safety Council, 1991), 2.

33. "Connections: 1992 Member Services Guide" (American Dental Association, Chicago, 1992), 4.

34. *EMOA-4*, 269.

35. "American Optometric Association: A Look Behind the Logo" (American Optometric Association, St. Louis, Mo., 1992, Brochure).

36. National Safety Council, *Looking Toward Tomorrow*, 14–15.

37. Ibid., 5–6.

38. "The American Red Cross: People Helping People" (American National Red Cross, Washington, D.C., 1989, Brochure).

39. *EMOA-4*, 859.

40. *EMOA-4*, 546.

41. *EMOA-3*, 373.

42. *Encyclopedia of Associations*, 23rd ed. (Detroit: Gale Research, 1989), 1344.

43. Letter from Jennifer C. Wellman, National Center for Homeopathy, to the author, 3 April 1992.

44. "American College of Cardiology 1992 Fact Sheet" (American College of Cardiology, Bethesda, Md., 1992).
45. *EMOA-4*, 884.
46. *EMOA-4*, 967.
47. Letter from Cynthia G. Swank to Joan Krizack, 19 Oct. 1992.
48. *EMOA-2*, 96. This organization is not listed in the third or fourth editions.
49. *EMOA-4*, 4.
50. Feldstein, *Health Associations*, 27. In 1965 the AMA spent more money opposing Medicare during the first three months of the year than any other lobbying organization spent during the entire year!
51. Feldstein, *Health Associations*, passim.
52. *EMOA-4*, 4.
53. *EMOA-4*, 269.
54. *EMOA-4*, 644.
55. *EMOA-4*, 544.
56. *EMOA-4*, 859.
57. Letter from Cynthia G. Swank to Joan Krizack, 19 Oct. 1992.
58. American Heart Association, *American Heart Association History 1992* (Dallas, Tex.: American Heart Association, 1992), 14.
59. National Safety Council, *Looking Toward Tomorrow*, 13.
60. *The First Ten Years: Gay Men's Health Crisis 1990–1991 Annual Report* (New York: Gay Men's Health Crisis, 1992), 3–7.
61. Planned Parenthood Federation of America, *A Tradition of Choice: 1991 Service Report* (New York: Planned Parenthood Federation of America, 1991), 5.
62. American National Red Cross, *The American Red Cross Biomedical Research and Development Report, 1991* (Washington, D.C.: American National Red Cross, 1991).
63. *EMOA-4*, 649.
64. "American College of Cardiology Organizational Chart for Board and Committees" (American College of Cardiology, Bethesda, Md., 1991).
65. "American Heart Association of Metropolitan Chicago Organizational Structure" (American Heart Association of Metropolitan Chicago, Chicago, 1991).
66. *EMOA-4*, 71.
67. *EMOA-4*, 459.
68. *EMOA-4*, 643.
69. *EMOA-4*, 23.
70. *EMOA-4*, 22.
71. *EMOA-4*, 415.
72. *EMOA-4*, 19.
73. *EMOA-4*, 7.
74. Letter from Linda Hudson, Vice President for Communications, Illinois State Medical Society, to the author, 5 Feb. 1992. All information given about the Illinois State Medical Society in this section is based on material provided by the society itself.
75. This development coincided almost exactly with the founding of the

American College of Cardiology (ACC) in 1949; the ACC and AHA now have a number of joint committees and task forces.

76. American Heart Association, *History 1992*, 1. All information about the AHA in this section is drawn from recent publications provided by the association itself.

77. American Heart Association, *History 1992*, 6.

78. Ibid.

79. The single voluntary association represented is the American Alliance of Health, Physical Education, Recreation and Dance, headquartered in Reston, Virginia.

80. Part of the rationale for this procedure is that the Sophia Smith Collection also holds the papers of early birth control advocate and Planned Parenthood founder Margaret Sanger.

81. AMA Archives staff are also responsible for answering public inquiries on current AMA policies, so the proportion of time devoted to archival functions is lower than the 1 FTE figure might suggest. In addition, as of November 1993 the AMA was engaged in significant cutbacks of its library and archival operations, so this description of the archives' operations may soon be outdated.

82. This figure presumably excludes the incumbent's salary and benefits.

83. It should be noted, however, that AIDS documentation projects are being carried out at the University of California at San Francisco and by volunteer archivists Kathryn Hammond Baker, Stanley Moss, and Nancy Richard at AIDS Action Committee in Boston.

84. Gay Men's Health Crisis reports that in 1991 it distributed exactly 1,468,256 such pieces (as well as 1,342,317 condoms). One hopes that, at least, GMHC is preserving sample copies of its literature, as well as the periodic "AIDS Fact Sheet" from which the above statistics are drawn.

85. However, the Gay Men's Health Crisis has successfully negotiated with the New York Public Library to house their records.

86. The sources consulted include the National Union Catalog of Manuscript Collections (NUCMC) and the online databases of the Research Libraries Information Network (RLIN) and Online Computer Library Center (OCLC). The total of 130 excludes duplicate entries for the same collection in more than one source.

87. A very high proportion of these records represent New York State and are held by the New York Academy of Medicine; the Downstate Medical Center, Brooklyn; and the Cornell University Archives. Probably there are other states whose medical societies are comparably well documented but that have not benefited from grant funding to support the entry of cataloging information into national databases, as has been the case in New York.

SELECT ANNOTATED BIBLIOGRAPHY

There appears to be no single book-length treatment of the history and role of health care associations, either professional or voluntary. A brief overview of the subject appears in James M. Rosser and Howard E. Mossberg, *An Analysis of Health Care Delivery* (New York: John Wiley & Sons, 1977), 29–35. For an article-length treatment of a single specialty see Bertram Slaff, "History of Child and Adolescent Psychiatry Ideas and Organizations in the United States: A Twentieth-Century Review," *Adolescent Psychiatry* 16 (1989): 31–52.

The legislative lobbying activities of selected health associations, including the American Medical Association, American Dental Association, American Nurses' Association, and American Hospital Association, are treated in Paul J. Feldstein, *Health Associations and the Demand for Legislation: The Political Economy of Health* (Cambridge, Mass.: Ballinger, 1977).

The American Medical Association has been the subject of at least three book-length historical works, namely James G. Burrow, *AMA: Voice of American Medicine* (Baltimore: Johns Hopkins Press, 1963), Frank D. Campion, *The AMA and U.S. Health Policy Since 1940* (Chicago: Chicago Review Press, 1984); and Morris Fishbein, *A History of the American Medical Association, 1847 to 1947* (Philadelphia: W. B. Saunders Co. 1947).

The field is littered with histories of state, local, and specialty societies, of variable quality and length. A small and arbitrary sample includes James Gilliam Hughes, *American Academy of Pediatrics: The First 50 Years* (Evanston, Ill.: American Academy of Pediatrics, 1980); Joseph Roy Jones, *History of the Medical Society of the State of California* (Sacramento: Historical Committee of the Sacramento Society for Medical Improvement, 1964); and Leonard A. Lewis, "The History of the American Society for Dermatologic Surgery and Its Impact on the Specialty of Dermatology," *Journal of Dermatologic Surgery and Oncology* 16, no. 11 (1990): 1054–56.

Among voluntary associations, the American Cancer Society seems to be unique in having been the subject of a book-length history: Walter Sanford Ross, *Crusade: The Official History of the American Cancer Society* (New York: Arbor House, ca. 1987). A few articles (again, greatly varied in both length and quality) have been devoted specifically to archives and archival activities of health organizations. These include T. A. Appel, "The Archives of the American Physiological Society," *Physiologist* 27, no.3 (1984), 131–32; Linda Cox, Geraldine Hutner, and Robin Kennett, "Creating the Archives," *New Jersey Medicine* 85, no. 9 (1985), 734–53; Robert S. Sparkman, "The Collection and Preservation of the Archives of the Southern Surgical Association," *Annals of Surgery* 207, no. 5 (1988), 533–37; and Manfred Waserman, "A Catalogue of the Manuscripts and Archives of the Library of the College of Physicians of Philadelphia, by Rudolf Hirsch" [essay review], *Transactions and Studies of the College of Physicians of Philadelphia* 5, no. 4 (1983), 385–87.

The standard reference on current health associations and organizations is *Encyclopedia of Medical Organizations and Agencies*, 4th ed. (Detroit: Gale Research, 1992).

CHAPTER 7

Health Industries

Providing the goods and services that support the U.S. health care system is the principal function of one of the largest and most profitable components of the U.S. health care system, the health industries. This "medical industrial complex," as it has been labeled,[1] supports the other components of the health care system by inventing, developing, and distributing such goods as drugs and medical equipment and by providing a broad range of services from laundering to computing. The health industries not only provide the foundation of the health care system, but also are a dominant force in the world of corporate America. In 1991 five of the twenty-five most profitable U.S. companies were in the health industries.[2]

The for-profit nature of most of the health industries sets them apart from the other institutions and organizations examined in this book. Like other components of the U.S. health care system, these industries play a significant role in helping people—saving lives and improving the quality of life. Because these industries are driven by the profit motive, however, the emphasis on getting a better product or service to market faster and with as low an overhead as possible is the measure of success and even of survival. This chapter examines the for-profit industries that compose the medical industrial complex.[3]

Health industries can be broadly grouped into two categories: those that manufacture and distribute goods to the medical marketplace and those that provide health-related services to physicians, hospitals, other health care providers, and the general consumer. The two major types of manufacturers and distributors of health care goods are pharmaceutical companies, and medical supplies and equipment companies. Pharmaceutical companies, such as Eli Lilly and Company, Merck & Co., and Bristol-Myers Squibb, develop and manufacture drugs and related products and deliver and provide support for these goods. Medical supplies and equipment manufacturers, such as Johnson & Johnson (which also manufactures pharmaceuticals) and Baxter International, are responsible for the design, manufacture, delivery, and support of a wide range of products, including surgical and medical instruments, x-ray equipment, contact lenses, and snakebite kits. A third type of industry, often overlooked in examinations of the medical industrial complex but of significant importance in the delivery and support of health care in the late twentieth century, is medical publishing. Medical publishers range from companies that publish in all disciplines, such as McGraw-Hill, to companies that focus solely on scientific and medical literature, such as Gower Medical Publishing. Academic and association presses are other important players in medical publishing, but they are often less profit driven than the commercial publishing houses.

The service segment of the health industries is vast. The largest and most influential service industry in the United States is the health insurance industry. By the late 1980s over 86 percent of the civilian population in the United States (more than 205 million Americans) was protected by one or more forms of health care insurance. Health insurance companies are a large part of the profit-making segment of the U.S. health care system. Other types of service industries include firms that support the health industries and other elements of the health care system, such as drug testing companies, which perform clinical trials for pharmaceutical manufacturers, and private independent laboratories, which perform analyses for hospitals and physicians. Health care industries that provide services also include a broad array of other enterprises such as hospital management firms, food services, laundry services, computing centers, and architecture and building consultants. An example of a service industry is ARA Services, which started as a supplier of vending machines in hospital waiting rooms and is now one of the largest food service companies in the United States as well as a leading provider of uniforms, linens, and other services to hospitals and nursing homes. Another example is American Medical Buildings, which develops, designs, and supervises construction of medical buildings and clinics.

This chapter examines the largest sector within each of the two broad categories of health industries, the goods providers and the service providers. Pharmaceutical companies are examined as an example of a goods manufacturing industry; the medical supplies and equipment industry and medical publishing are examined in less detail. In the service sector, the health insurance industry is discussed. The examination of pharmaceutical companies and health insurance providers begins with a historical overview of each industry, providing a foundation for discussing the industry's functions. These functions are explored, and similarities and differences are highlighted.

PHARMACEUTICAL COMPANIES

The pharmaceutical industry, considered the most profitable major manufacturing sector since the late nineteenth century, is a large and powerful component of the U.S. economy and of the U.S. health care system's health industries.[4] There are over 500 pharmaceutical manufacturers in the United States and several have annual sales of over $5 billion, led in 1991 by Bristol-Myers Squibb, with sales over $11 billion, and Merck & Co., with sales of $8.6 billion. Merck and Bristol-Myers Squibb also ranked fourth and fifth in total profits for all U.S. corporations in 1991.[5]

TYPES OF PHARMACEUTICAL COMPANIES

Pharmaceutical companies can be classified into four broad groupings according to the type of drugs they produce and how the drugs are distributed. These groupings are[6]:

- ethical companies
- "over-the-counter" (OTC) companies
- generic companies
- "start-up" biotechnology and experimental companies

As for other aspects of the health industries, the distinctions between these groups have blurred in recent years. Companies that originally focused on one type of drug have broadened their focus to include other types.

Ethical companies are research-based drug companies that market their products to health care providers and delivery facilities. The term "ethical" was first used in the early twentieth century and was meant to denote honest. It subsequently came to apply to medicines that were not publicly advertised.[7] Examples of ethical companies are Eli Lilly and Company, Merck & Co., and the Upjohn Company. OTC companies are marketing-based companies that sell products directly to the consumer. Bristol-Myers Squibb and Warner-Lambert are examples of OTC companies (although both also have prescription drug divisions). Generic companies also are marketing-based companies which on patent expiration convert proprietary products to generic drugs and sell them to health care providers and delivery facilities. Examples of these companies are Mylan Laboratories, Quad Pharmaceuticals, and Bolar Pharmaceutical Company. The biotechnology and experimental companies within the pharmaceutical industry are research-based companies that use new techniques, in particular genetic engineering and structure-based design, to develop new products. Amgen, Biogen, and Vertex are examples of these types of companies.

HISTORY

Some pharmaceutical companies have their roots in centuries-old traditions. Merck & Co., for example, traces its antecedents to 1668, when Friedrich Jacob Merck purchased an apothecary in Darmstadt, Germany.[8] Several American firms started in the first half of the nineteenth century, and many others were founded later in the 1800s. The history of the pharmaceutical industry itself, however, is little more than a century old, its growth and development coinciding with the rise of scientific medicine in the late nineteenth century and the simultaneous emergence of entrepreneurial tendencies in the U.S. health care system. The formation of the American pharmaceutical industry was influenced by such factors as the public health movements of the period, initial efforts at government regulation, scientific breakthroughs such as the discovery of salvarsan (used in the treatment of protozoan infections), changes in the educational system that produced scientists to work in this growing economy, and even the chain drugstore movement.

Some scholars argue that the pharmaceutical industry did not evolve into its modern form until World War II, when the focus of the industry shifted from drug manufacturing to drug innovation. This transformation took place in part because of the discovery of the therapeutic powers of drugs such as the sulfonamides in the 1930s and the increased demand for drugs during World War II. After penicillin was released for civilian use in 1945, the rate of drug innovation increased dramatically. The first half of the 1940s saw 67 new drugs introduced into the U.S. market; by the last half of the 1950s, this number had reached 248.[9]

The history of the pharmaceutical industry following World War II is dominated by a rapid increase in scientific research and development efforts, but other factors also played large roles. One factor was governmental regulation of therapeutic drug manufacturing. Although governmental control of drugs generally dates back to the 1906 Pure Food and Drug Act, the focus of the 1906 act was largely on food adulteration and abuse and less on drug regulation.[10] It was not until 1938, when a new Food, Drug, and Cosmetic Act was passed, that more emphasis was placed on drug regulation. The 1938 act, a result in part of the deaths associated with inadequately tested new drugs such as sulfanilamide, called for premarketing testing of drugs. However, this legislation failed to provide an adequate regulatory agency, as the legal powers of the Food and Drug Administration (FDA) were considered "somewhat ambiguous."[11] It was not until the early 1960s when another tragedy, precipitated by the use of thalidomide, led to the strengthening of the regulatory powers of the 1938 act.[12] The 1962 amendments "empowered the FDA to specify the testing procedure a manufacturer must use to produce acceptable information for evaluating the NDA [new drug application]."[13] These amendments also required for the first time that manufacturers provide proof of the efficacy as well as safety of new drugs. Although the 1962 amendments have left a trail of controversy in the thirty years since their passage, they have continued to serve as the basis for drug regulatory actions. In the 1980s, largely as a result of the acquired immunodeficiency syndrome (AIDS) epidemic, substantial rethinking of the federal regulatory role and of specific policies was initiated and certain changes were proposed. One result was that in May 1987, the FDA adopted a new rule that allowed the release of experimental drugs to individuals with AIDS and other serious diseases before final approval of the drugs. Azidothymidine (AZT), shown to be an effective drug against the human immunodeficiency virus, was one of the first drugs released in this manner.[14]

Governmental control of the release of new drugs is not the only aspect of regulation that is significant in the pharmaceutical industry. The FDA has also become increasingly involved in economic aspects of the pharmaceutical industry, including pricing, marketing, and competition. The Federal Trade Commission monitors economic aspects of the pharmaceutical industry, such as the industry's high return on equity and also controls the advertising of OTC drugs.[15]

These concerns about the pharmaceutical industry highlight another major area of the development of the industry in the post–World War II period: economic growth and the competition, diversification, and consolidation that resulted from this growth. The extent of this growth can be demonstrated in a number of ways but perhaps none more dramatic than the seventeenfold increase in sales of prescription drugs in the thirty years following the end of World War II. In addition to the fact that there were more drugs in the marketplace as a result of effective research and development efforts, events such as the passage of Medicare and Medicaid legislation in the mid-1960s made it easier and often cheaper for Americans to receive drug treatment. Increased advertising, especially on television, contributed to this growth in drug sales. Even cultural and societal changes, ranging from such factors as an increase in stressful white collar

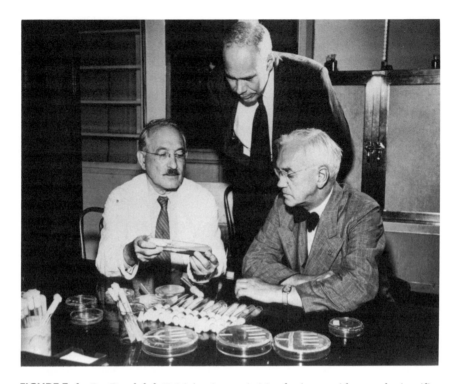

FIGURE 7-1   Dr. Randolph T. Major (center), Merck vice president and scientific director, meets in 1949 with Dr. Selman A. Waksman (left), in whose Rutgers University laboratory streptomycin was discovered, and with Sir Alexander Fleming, nobel laureate and discoverer of penicillin. *Source:* Merck & Co., Inc., Whitehouse Station, N.J.

occupations to the civil, political, and social upheavals that affected Americans in the postwar decades, may have played a part in the economic growth of the industry. As Walter Measday noted in 1977, "It may be a commentary on our society that shipments of tranquilizers alone today exceed the entire output of the industry in 1939 by a wide margin."[16]

The industry's growth led to significant and often brutal competition. According to David Schwartzman, two competitive strategies are available to a pharmaceutical manufacturer: cutting prices or seeking innovations.[17] Both tactics have been used in the pharmaceutical industry over the past forty years to obtain a larger market share and to seek a more favorable profit margin.

The economic growth of the pharmaceutical industry also led to diversification and consolidation among companies involved in producing drugs for the U.S. health care system. In similar fashion to other components of the U.S. health care system, pharmaceutical companies have increasingly become economically and organizationally parts of larger institutions dealing with a variety of products and services. The Upjohn Company had its origins in the late nineteenth century as the Upjohn Pill and Granule Company with the manufacture of pills as its primary focus. However, like other long-standing American drug-producing firms such as Lilly and SmithKline, in the post-1950 period Upjohn began to diversify into such areas as agricultural and aerospace products. The diversification at Lilly, which began pill manufacturing in 1876, included agricultural products, which by the 1980s accounted for 30% of sales, and cosmetics, which represented 10% of sales.[18] In the late twentieth century, other leading research-based drug manufacturers, such as American Home Products, emerged as pharmaceutical giants after years of producing a variety of other consumer products, some of which were health related. In another aspect of economic diversification, the leading pharmaceutical companies have become international in scope, combining with established foreign companies or extending their own sales and manufacturing operations beyond U.S. boundaries.

The development of the pharmaceutical industry in the twentieth century focuses on research, innovation, and the swift delivery of products to the marketplace. In these characteristics, it is similar to the other health industries discussed in this chapter. Similarly, the impact of regulatory agencies on health industries has become a major factor in the post–World War II period. All these factors have an impact on the profitability of these industries, which is, of course, the most critical measure of their success.

HEALTH INDUSTRY FUNCTIONS

As noted at the outset of this chapter, the primary function of the health industries in the U.S. health care system is the provision of goods and services (see Table 7-1), which is composed of several activities: research and development, marketing and sales, and production and distribution. In addition, certain health industries are minimally involved in the health promotion function and all engage in institutional administration.[19] (See Table 7-2.) Most of these functions comprise specific activities within each type of health industry, and these are discussed below. Institutional administration, which is common to all the health industries, is discussed briefly here for the sake of convenience. Although the discussion is brief, the importance of the administration function in the health industries should not be overlooked.

TABLE 7–1 Role of health industries in the U.S. health care system

	Functions of the U.S. Health Care System					
	Health Care Delivery					
Industry	Patient Care	Health Promotion	Biomedical Research	Education	Regulation/ Policy Formulation	Provision of Goods/ Services
Pharmaceutical companies	2		1			1
Medical supplies/ equipment manufacturers	2		2			1
Medical publish- ing companies						1
Health insurance companies	2					1

1 = primary function, 2 = secondary function.

TABLE 7-2 Institutional Functions of Health Industries

Industry	Research and Development	Marketing and Sales	Production and Distribution	Corporate Management	Health Promotion
Pharmaceutical companies	1	1	1	1	2
Medical supplies/ equipment manufacturers	1	1	1	1	2
Medical publishing companies		1	1	1	
Health insurance companies		1	1	1	2

1 = primary function, 2 = secondary function.

CORPORATE MANAGEMENT IN THE HEALTH INDUSTRIES

As expected with for-profit businesses, the function of corporate management is a major one in the health industries. The principal activities within this function include:

- governance
- fiscal management
- personnel management
- operations management
- facilities management
- external relations

The nature and extent of each activity within each health industry depend on the product or service, the size of the industry, and such factors as the role of the industry in relation to broader corporate structures (e.g., parent companies, subsidiaries, etc.).

FUNCTIONS OF THE PHARMACEUTICAL INDUSTRY

In addition to the common function of institutional administration noted above, the pharmaceutical industry is involved in research and development, marketing and sales, production and distribution, and health promotion. Each of these functions is examined below.

Research and Development in the Pharmaceutical Industry   As is evident from the historical overview provided earlier, research is a critical function of the pharmaceutical industry. It is, in effect, the lifeblood of the industry. In many ways, the research efforts of pharmaceutical companies are at the center of patient care in the United States. As Schnee and Caglarian noted, "The primary purpose of pharmaceutical research is to aid in the prevention, diagnosis, and treatment of disease and general promotion of health."[20] Three specific activities are included within the research function in the pharmaceutical industry: research, testing, and regulatory submission and approval.

Research   Pharmaceutical companies are involved in both basic and applied drug research.[21] In the past two decades, the trend has been to focus less on basic research and more on applied research.[22] Part of the reason for this development is that the costs of basic research have skyrocketed since the 1960s, and the financial return on investment in basic research has not been as great as in the two decades following World War II. Another reason for the decline in basic research activity is that there is a limit to the new drugs that can be discovered. New chemical entities, the essence of new drug discoveries, are rare, and after the surge of discovery and development in the 1940s and 1950s (when over 3,500 new products and dosage forms were introduced) it became necessary to move into other areas of innovation. Such areas include development of duplicate products, compounded products, and alternate dosage forms.[23] In the 1970s and 1980s, pharmaceutical companies increasingly put a greater emphasis on these latter categories of drug innovation.

Testing   In all types of drug research, a wide range of methods of drug testing is undertaken, including toxicology tests and clinical studies. Although most drug research takes place within pharmaceutical companies at their own expense, some aspects of this testing, such as clinical trials (the investigation of the effects of a drug administered to human subjects), are undertaken on contract by laboratories and other for-profit organizations outside the companies. As noted in Chapter 4, a number of multimillion dollar contracts between academic medical centers and pharmaceutical companies were signed in the 1980s. In fact, the pharmaceutical industry has a substantial history of cooperative research with American universities, beginning in the 1920s and 1930s with such collaborative efforts as those between Abbott Laboratories and pharmacologists at the University of Wisconsin.[24]

Regulatory Submission and Approval   Drug testing within the pharmaceutical companies is a direct result of regulatory stipulations placed on these companies by federal legislation. Thus the activity of preparing a new drug for submission to the FDA is an integral activity. The process of regulation does not apply only to the actual submission of a proposed new drug; governmental controls also exist for most aspects of premarketing testing, from preclinical (animal) to clinical testing. The entire process of bringing a drug to market, from innovation to marketing, is tightly woven with regulatory guidelines and mandates.

Marketing and Sales in the Pharmaceutical Industry   In the pharmaceutical industry, the marketing and sales function is composed of the separate activities of marketing research and planning, advertising, and sales (or, in the industry's terminology, detailing).[25] A study by the Congressional Office of Technology Assessment found that the pharmaceutical industry's marketing and advertising costs average about $10 billion per year.[26]

Marketing Research and Planning   Marketing research and planning is in itself a business within the business of the pharmaceutical industry.

Pharmaceutical companies as well as outside firms undertake extensive research and analysis of physician needs and prescribing behavior, which provides information used to devise strategies to develop and market products.[27]

Advertising   Advertising is key to the marketing strategies of pharmaceutical companies. Several hundred million dollars are expended annually in the United States on drug advertising. Again, depending on the type of company, the nature and extent of advertising varies. Ethical companies traditionally have advertised strictly to health care providers, primarily through professional journals. In recent years, appeals by ethical companies aimed directly at lay consumers have appeared in television and magazine advertising, the method most often used by OTC companies. These ads, however, generally are not for specific products but are used to promote corporate visibility and goodwill for the industry. Some medical publishers, returning to tactics used in the nineteenth century, are producing books that contain pharmaceutical advertising interspersed with the text.[28] Free samples distributed to physicians and then passed on to patients are used not only as a form of informal clinical evaluation of a product but also as an effective means of promoting the product. Expenditures for samples approximate those for journal advertising among the leading pharmaceutical companies. Other promotional campaigns, such as giveaways of pens, pads, and notebooks advertising the company and its products, are also used by the pharmaceutical companies. In recent years the FDA and several medical societies have sought to place restrictions on these giveaways.[29]

Sales (Detailing)   Depending on the type of pharmaceutical company (see Types of Pharmaceutical Companies, above), the scope of sales varies, but the focus is generally the same: introducing new products, new dosages, and new medical uses as well as selling existing products. Pharmaceutical companies employ sales representatives to call on physicians, hospital pharmacists, wholesalers, and other health care providers. Companies also use direct mail campaigns, telemarketing, and, of course, media advertising to sell their products.

Production and Distribution in the Pharmaceutical Industry   Production of goods in the pharmaceutical industry is largely driven by the two functions of research and development and marketing and sales. After new products are developed and approved, production is the next step. The role of marketing and sales, however, plays an equally (and some might argue more) important role in production of goods. In a for-profit corporation, the demand for the product (often largely influenced by marketing and sales activity) clearly guides production. Consequently, the general function of corporate management comes into play in the production process as the various activities of fiscal management, materials management, and even plant management may determine production quotas and directions.

Distribution of products in the pharmaceutical industry depends on the type of company involved. Ethical companies distribute primarily to health care providers, whereas OTC companies focus on consumers. In each case, wholesalers play an important role as the conduit for indirect drug sales.

Health Promotion in the Pharmaceutical Industry   "The business of the drug industry is human health," as David Siskind noted in 1978,[30] and therefore health promotion is an integral function of pharmaceutical companies, although one that is of less importance than the other functions discussed earlier in this chapter. Insofar as much of the focus of the pharmaceutical industry is on health care providers, the preponderance of health promotion by the industry is directed toward physicians and others who decide what drugs should be used. Thus, health promotion in the pharmaceutical industry is largely an "educational effort" (the preferred term of the industry) aimed at practicing physicians.[31] Most of this "education" takes place in the advertising and sales effort of the companies. Nevertheless, promotional advertisements directed at consumers have begun to appear on television and in magazines. In addition, some pharmaceutical companies, in response to the rise in drug abuse and the AIDS epidemic, are sponsoring promotional campaigns tied in to increasing public awareness of these issues.

MEDICAL SUPPLIES AND EQUIPMENT MANUFACTURERS

Medical supplies and equipment manufacturing is a large and diverse component of the medical industrial complex. The spectrum of products generated by this industry ranges from Band-Aids to high technology equipment. The 1976 Medical Device Amendments (Public Law 94–295) to the Federal Food, Drug, and Cosmetic Act defined a medical device as "any instrument, apparatus, or similar or related article that is intended to prevent, diagnose, mitigate, or treat disease or to affect the structure or function of the body."[32]

The range of this industry is vast. Nearly 3,000 manufacturing establishments are registered with the Bureau of Medical Devices of the FDA, and these companies produce items that fall into more than 160 Standard Industrial Classification codes. The bulk of these products fall into six major categories: surgical and medical instruments; surgical appliances and supplies, dental equipment and supplies, x-ray apparatus and tubes, electromedical equipment, and ophthalmic goods.[33]

In 1991 three companies dominated the sales in the U.S. medical supplies and equipment market—Johnson & Johnson, with $12.4 billion in sales, Baxter International, with $8.9 billion, and Abbott Laboratories, with $6.8 billion. Johnson & Johnson also was the fourteenth highest profit earning company in 1991 and of the top twenty-five corporations in profit earnings had the largest percentage increase in profit from 1990 to 1991 (28 percent).[34]

MEDICAL SUPPLIES AND EQUIPMENT MANUFACTURERS' FUNCTIONS

The functions of medical supplies and equipment manufacturers are similar to those of the pharmaceutical companies. Research and development, marketing and sales, and production and distribution are the primary functions; health promotion is a secondary function. Although the medical supplies and equipment manufacturers do not undertake biomedical research as do the pharmaceutical companies, they do rely on research in such areas as engineering and product development to strengthen their position in the marketplace and bring marketable products to consumers as quickly as possible. As in the pharmaceutical industry, competition is keen in the areas of innovation and product delivery. Regulatory submission and approval, although not as stringent as in the pharmaceutical industry, still play a major role in the medical supplies and equipment industry. Within the marketing and sales function, activities similar to those of the pharmaceutical industry can be found in medical supplies and equipment manufacturers. Marketing research and planning, advertising, and sales are important. Production is driven by market needs and corporate directions. Distribution and support services are a large part of the industry, with the support service aspect being perhaps more prominent in the medical equipment industry than in the pharmaceutical industry, owing to the need for technical support for equipment and other devices. As with the pharmaceutical companies, health promotion in the form of "educating" is a function of the medical supplies and equipment industry, which similarly targets the health care providers to whom products are sold.

MEDICAL PUBLISHING

Recording medical advances, knowledge, and information is an aspect of the U.S. health care system as old as the profession itself. The industry of medical publishing might be said to date from the eighteenth century when publishers of medical journals first appeared regularly in Europe although scientific and medical books had been published for centuries. In the two centuries since that time, medical publishing has become a critical and central part of the U.S. health care system. After World War II, and especially beginning in the 1960s, the volume of medical publishing increased at a dramatic rate. The information explosion characteristic of other fields was no less evident in health care. Expansion of the medical publishing industry to include data base creation and distribution is a phenomenon of the computer revolution, and the National Library of Medicine's production of MEDLINE in the 1960s was one of the earliest developments in this area. CD-ROM publications first appeared in the 1980s, and the first electronic medical journal appeared in 1992.[35]

The two dominant functions of the medical publishing industry are the marketing and sales and the production and distribution of goods. Unlike the other industries examined thus far, there is no direct involvement in research or health promotion. The publishing industry's goods, however, are indispensable to the operation of the U.S. health care system as a whole and to research in particular.

INSURANCE COMPANIES

The health insurance industry, like the other health industries discussed in this chapter, is a big business in America. Joseph Califano, in his analysis of the "profitable acolytes" of American health care, remarked that "the commercial insurance companies and the Blues are the money changers, particularly in the temples of hospital care."[36] Two U.S. health insurance companies, Aetna Life & Casualty and CIGNA, had sales in excess of $18 billion in 1991.[37]

TYPES OF HEALTH INSURANCE

There are four predominant forms of health insurance coverage in the United States:[38]

- private for-profit (commercial insurance companies)
- private nonprofit (Blue Cross and Blue Shield)

- nonprofit prepayment plans (HMOs, PPOs)
- government funded programs (Medicare and Medicaid)

Within these types of insurance providers there are four basic types of health insurance:

- hospitalization
- surgery
- regular medical expenses
- major medical expenses

Hospitalization insurance includes normal and necessary hospital expenses such as the cost of the hospital room and meals, use of the operating room, x-ray and laboratory fees, and some medicines and supplies. Surgical insurance covers the cost of operations, up to certain limits. Regular medical expense policies also pay for doctors' services other than surgical treatment, either in the hospital or elsewhere. Major medical policies protect the insured against catastrophic charges, generally paying most costs—up to a total ranging from $10,000 to as much as $250,000—above an initial deductible amount that is paid by the policy holder.[39]

HISTORY

Despite the tremendous volume of business in the health insurance industry, the industry itself is a relatively recent development on the American health care scene. Although there are nineteenth-century precedents for health insurance coverage, primarily associated with fraternal orders and industries such as lumber and mining, health insurance on an individual or national basis was not widely accepted or desired in the nineteenth century. The American Medical Association (AMA), in fact, long condemned the concept of "contract practices."[40] The passage of a National Insurance Act in Great Britain in 1911, combined with increasing costs for medical care, caused Americans in the Progressive Era to become interested in compulsory health insurance. For a variety of reasons, however, including wavering support from the AMA and U.S. involvement in World War I, interest in compulsory health insurance had largely subsided by the end of the second decade of the century. By 1925 the New York State Medical Society reported that health insurance was "a dead issue in the United States."[41]

Although the spirit of compulsory health insurance was subdued for over a decade, the basis for a revival in interest in and support for health insurance continued to develop. From the 1910s to the 1940s, workmen's compensation was the most common form of health insurance in America and helped to keep the notion of some type of medical assistance alive. The Depression years of the 1930s created the appropriate mood for addressing the issue of health insurance for workers and the needy. During these years several hospitals began experimenting with hospital prepayment or insurance plans. One of the most influential of these was the Baylor University Hospital plan, considered to be the precursor of the Blue Cross movement.[42] The success of the Baylor plan attracted the interest of other hospitals, and by 1937 twenty-six such plans were in operation. During that year the American Hospital Association and the AMA's House of Delegates began approving such plans, and the Health Service Plan Commission (later the Blue Cross Commission) was organized.

In the late 1930s surgical-medical plans were also being developed; the first was the California Physicians Service in 1939. This led to the organization in 1946 of the Blue Shield Medical Care Plans, Inc. (later Blue Shield Commission). Even the AMA became supportive of health insurance and created its own Associated Medical Care Plan. The medical profession had come to see the advantages of health insurance, particularly the economic ones (e.g., regular payments). A key step forward for health insurance came through litigation when in 1948 the Supreme Court ruled that health insurance benefits could be included in collective bargaining.

By the early 1950s, a majority of Americans had purchased health insurance of some type.[43] From the 1950s to the mid-1960s, the health insurance industry saw continuous growth. In the mid-1960s, the health insurance industry, as well as the health care industry as a whole, changed even more dramatically with the enactment of Medicare and Medicaid legislation. As Ronald Numbers points out, "In 1967, just two years after the passage of Medicare, third parties for the first time paid more than half of the nation's medical bills."[44] This historic watershed set the stage for further growth of the health insurance industry as it developed into a multibillion dollar institution in the following decades.

From the late 1970s to the late 1980s the health insurance market changed significantly. In the 1970s the marketplace was dominated by commercial insurers and Blue Cross/Blue Shield plans. A decade later the predominance of commercial insurers and the "Blues" had been eroded by the fact that many employers were self-insured and by the significant growth of preferred provider organizations and health maintenance organizations. One result of this change in the health insurance market was increased competition among health insurers. This trend is likely to foster further change in the health insurance industry in the coming decade, as is the rekindling of the debate over national health insurance.[45]

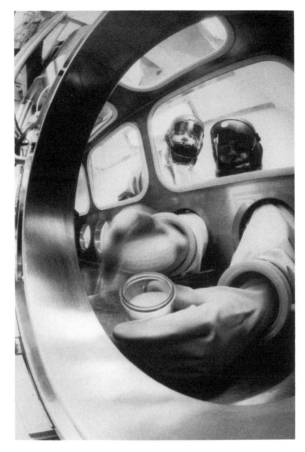

FIGURE 7–2   A group production manager (left) watches a process operator as he examines a sample of the active ingredient for PROSCAR, a drug for treating benign prostatic hyperplasia, in a sterile glove box, 1991. *Source:* Merck & Co., Inc., Whitehouse Station, N.J.

FUNCTIONS OF THE HEALTH INSURANCE INDUSTRY

The primary function of the health insurance industry in the U.S. health care system is to provide insurance coverage. The institutional functions within the health insurance industry are similar to those in the pharmaceutical and medical equipment and supply manufacturers, although the definition and dimensions of these functions differ in the service industry of health insurance.

Research and Development in the Health Insurance Industry

Much of the research done by insurance companies is sociological and economic (examining the demographics and statistics of the U.S. society and economy) rather than biomedical, as in the case of pharmaceutical companies. Although insurance companies are interested in basic research and sponsor significant amounts of such research, the type of research undertaken by the industry itself is largely applied. Other aspects of the research function, as discussed for the goods manufacturers, do not apply to the health insurance companies.

Marketing and Sales in the Health Insurance Industry

As with the pharmaceutical companies examined earlier, the marketing and sales function in the health insurance industry can be broken down into the separate activities of

- marketing research and planning
- advertising
- sales

Marketing research and planning in the health insurance industry, as noted above, center largely on sociological and economic areas. As with the pharmaceutical companies, this activity is a business in itself. Advertising is a major activity of the health insurance companies, although, because of increasing participation in group plans, direct advertising to the consumer for health insurance is not as prominent as with other types of insurance coverage (e.g., automobile insurance). Sales in the health insurance industry generally follow along the lines of sales in the other industries discussed earlier. The difference is that a large portion of the insurance covering Americans is not sold directly to the consumer but is marketed through employers or outgroup buyers. Although the insurance salesperson remains a fixture of American society, the emphasis of these individuals has shifted away from health insurance to other types of insurance coverage (such as life, automobile, and mortgage insurance).

Production and Distribution in the Health Insurance Industry

As a service industry, insurance involves no production of goods, distinguishing this industry from the pharmaceutical and medical suppliers and equipment manufacturers. Distribution and support services in the health insurance industry include such activities as claims reviews and processing of payments.

Health Promotion in the Health Insurance Industry Health insurance companies play a strong role in health promotion, as it is in their best interest that their clients remain healthy. Primarily as an offshoot to advertising and marketing campaigns, health insurance companies produce items, such as pamphlets on industrial safety and video tapes on child care, as a way to make the public aware of good health practices as well as of the services the insurance companies offer.

RECORDS OF HEALTH INDUSTRIES

As noted at the outset of this chapter, the for-profit nature of the health industries is an important characteristic of this segment of the U.S. health care system. It is also a dominant factor in the documentation issues within these industries. Documentation generated within any component of the U.S. health care system is preserved principally for purposes of recording the history and functions of the respective institutions. Within the health industries, however, the relationship of this documentation to the ongoing viability of the organization is more critical. Within the documentation generated by the health industries lies the very success (and potential failure, from a for-profit standpoint) of the organization.

Each function of the health industries, as examined in this chapter, produces records that hold varying degrees of corporate secrets, strategies, and perhaps skeletons. Issues such as corporate security and litigation present challenges to the maintenance and availability of these materials. The nature of the documentation, from fiscal records to research data, is sensitive and potentially a liability to the companies. The plethora of data gathered in the research process presents a dichotomous management situation. On the one hand, as Samuels pointed out in relation to the pharmaceutical companies, "The industry values information and recognizes the need for long-term access for scientific, regulatory, and management purposes."[46] On the other hand, these records are sensitive, for personal as well as corporate reasons, and close control of the documents is critical. Because of this, some companies may have initiated records retention policies that emphasize records destruction rather than records retention.[47] Such policies are counter to archival practices and, as early as the 1960s, led to a push among archivists for companies to retain company records chronicling the success and failures of a company's history.[48]

Largely as a result of this situation, the overall status of documenting the health industries is unclear. John Swann noted that "few drug companies maintain archives (or admit they do)."[49] An examination of the standard archival directories and reference tools supports Swann's assessment of the state of archives in the pharmaceutical industry as well as the other industries examined in this chapter.[50] The few entries that exist for the pharmaceutical industry in the Research Libraries Information Network (RLIN) are generally for the personal papers of researchers who worked for a leading pharmaceutical company, or pharmaceutical company records from the late nineteenth and early twentieth centuries that are now housed at a college or university. There are even fewer indications of records programs in the other health industries examined in this chapter. One interesting exception is that the records of several Silicon Valley medical equipment companies (predominantly "high tech" companies in such areas as medical imaging) are held at the Silicon Valley Information Center. These, too, however, are the "public records" of the companies, typically including press releases, quarterly and annual reports, and Securities and Exchange Commission (10-K) reports.[51]

On the positive side, a number of archivists or records managers in the health industries are listed in the *SAA Directory*. This seeming discrepancy only reaffirms the speculation that the industries examined here may have documentation programs in place but do not report such activities to the standard directories, largely for proprietary and business reasons. Without a thorough survey of the industries in question, a task beyond the scope of this study, it is difficult to assess the total nature of documentation. However, as with other components of the U.S. health care system, it is very likely that an increased documentation effort among the health industries is warranted.

NOTES

1. Stanley Wohl, *The Medical Industrial Complex* (New York: Harmony Books, 1984), 1.
2. "Corporate Scoreboard," *Business Week,* 16 March 1992, 65. The five companies are Merck & Co., Bristol-Myers Squibb, Johnson & Johnson, American Home Products, and Eli Lilly and Company.
3. Some types of health industries, notably health insurance providers such as Blue Cross/Blue Shield, are nonprofit and will not be discussed in detail here. On the other hand, portions of other institutions of the U.S. health care system are for-profit, such as some hospitals and nursing homes (see Chapter 2).
4. Jonathan Liebenau, *Medical Science and Medical Industry: The Formation of the American Pharmaceutical Industry* (Baltimore: Johns Hopkins University Press, 1987), vii.
5. D. J. De Rezno, ed., *Pharmaceutical Manufacturers in the United States* (Park Ridge, N.J.: Noyes Data, 1987), iii; "Corporate Scoreboard," *Business Week,* 16 March 1992, 65, 74.

202HEALTH INDUSTRIES

6. Helen W. Samuels, "Documenting Modern Chemistry: The Historical Task of the Archivist," (manuscript), 13–14.
7. (Liebenau, *Medical Science and Medical Industry*, 137, n. 18). This definition of ethical companies has changed in the 1990s as advertising aimed at the consumer has increasingly been used by traditional ethical companies. Still, the products are prescription drugs that are sold to pharmacies and not to the consumer.
8. Gary D. Nelson, *Pharmaceutical Company Histories*, vol. 1 (Bismarck, ND: Woodbine Publishing, 1983), 79.
9. Meir Statman, *Competition in the Pharmaceutical Industry: The Declining Profitability of Drug Innovation* (Washington, D.C.: American Enterprise Institute for Public Policy Research, 1983), 4–6.
10. Jerome E. Schnee, "Governmental Control of Therapeutic Drugs: Intent, Impact, and Issues," in Cotton M. Lindsay, ed., *The Pharmaceutical Industry: Economics, Performance, and Government Regulation* (New York: John Wiley & Sons, 1978), 9. For precedents to the 1906 act, see Mitchell Okun, *Fair Play in the Marketplace: The First Battle for Pure Food and Drugs* (DeKalb, Ill.: Northern Illinois University Press, 1986) and John B. Blake, ed., *Safeguarding the Public: Historical Aspects of Medicinal Drug Control* (Baltimore: Johns Hopkins Press, 1970).
11. Schnee, "Therapeutic Drugs," 10.
12. Thalidomide was found to cause severe malformations in limbs of developing fetuses. The impact of the thalidomide episode is chronicled by Henning Sjostrom and Robert Nilsson, *Thalidomide and the Power of the Drug Companies* (Baltimore: Penguin, 1972).
13. Schnee, "Therapeutic Drugs," 11.
14. Mary Graham, "The Quiet Drug Revolution," *Atlantic*, January 1991, 34–40.
15. Walter J. Campbell, "The Emerging Health Care Environment: Selected Issues," in Lindsay, *Pharmaceutical Industry*, 135–136.
16. Walter S. Measday, "The Pharmaceutical Industry," in Walter Adams, ed., *The Structure of American Industry*, 5th ed. (New York: Macmillan Publishing Co., 1977), 255.
17. David Schwartzman, *Innovation in the Pharmaceutical Industry* (Baltimore: Johns Hopkins University Press, 1976), 103.
18. Lilly's gross sales in 1985 were $3.27 billion, with $1.78 billion of that being pharmaceutical products. De Renzo, *Pharmaceutical Manufacturers*, 94. See also David Tucker, *The World Health Market: The Future of the Pharmaceutical Industry* (New York: Facts on File Publications, 1984), 24–25.
19. The categorization here is adopted from Califano, who characterizes the primary activities of the pharmaceutical companies as "to invent, patent, and market drugs," and Samuels, who lists the functions of the pharmaceutical companies as "research and development, testing of drugs, toxicology tests, clinical studies, regulatory submissions and approval, marketing and sales, corporate management." Joseph A. Califano, Jr., *America's Health Care Revolution: Who Lives? Who Dies? Who Pays?* (New York: Random House, 1986), 124; Samuels, "Documenting Modern Chemistry," 16–17.

20. Jerome E. Schnee and Erol Caglarian, "The Changing Pharmaceutical Research and Development Environment," in Lindsay, *Pharmaceutical Industry*, 91.
21. For a general discussion of the distinction between applied and basic research, see Chapter 4.
22. Schwartzman, *Pharmaecutical Industry*, 29.
23. Schnee and Caglarian, "Pharmaecutical Environment," 93.
24. John P. Swann, *Academic Scientists and the Pharmaceutical Industry: Cooperative Research in Twentieth-Century America* (Baltimore: Johns Hopkins University Press, 1988), 4.
25. Gilbert D. Harrell, "Pharmaceutical Marketing," in Lindsay, *Pharmaceutical Industry*, 69.
26. Constance Sommer, "Drug Firms Profits Exceed Other Industries, Report Says," *Boston Globe*, 26 Feb. 1993, 18. This figure is about $2 billion more than the industry spends annually to develop new drugs.
27. Harrell, "Pharmaceutical Marketing," 72.
28. See "Whittle and Drug Companies Team Up for Medical Books," *Publishers Weekly*, 17 May 1991, 44.
29. See Elisabeth Rosenthal, "Drug Companies' Profits Finance More Promotion Than Research," *New York Times*, 21 Feb. 1993, 1, 26.
30. David A. Siskind, "Contributions of the Pharmaceutical Industry to Improved Health," in Lindsay, *Pharmaceutical Industry*, 41.
31. Measday, "Pharmaecutical Industry," 269.
32. *Federal Policies and the Medical Device Industry* (Washington, D.C.: U.S. Congress, Office of Technology Assessment, OTA-H-230, October 1984), 4.
33. *1987 Census of Manufactures* (Washington, D.C.: U.S. Department of Commerce, Bureau of the Census, 1989), 1–2.
34. "Corporate Scoreboard," *Business Week*, 16 March 1992, 74, 65.
35. Mark Sexton, "AMPA and STM Discuss Medical Publishing Future," *Publishers Weekly*, 13 April 1990, 40; "First Electronic Medical Journal to Debut in 1992," *Library Journal* 1 Nov. 1991: 32.
36. Califano, *America's Health Care Revolution*, 124.
37. "Corporate Scoreboard," *Business Week*, 16 March 1992, 79.
38. *Source Book of Health Insurance Data, 1989* (Washington, D.C.: Health Insurance Association of America, [1989]), 7.
39. Malpractice insurance, which has played an increasingly large role in the economics of health care since World War II, is not treated here as "health insurance," but it is an important segment of the insurance industry and the U.S. health care system.
40. Ronald L. Numbers, "The Third Party: Health Insurance in America," in Judith Walzer Leavitt and Ronald L. Numbers, eds., *Sickness and Health in America: Readings in the History of Medicine and Public Health* (Madison: University of Wisconsin Press, 1978), 139.
41. Numbers, "Third Party," 139–141. Also see his *Almost Persuaded: American Physicians and Compulsory Health Insurance, 1912–1920* (Baltimore: Johns Hopkins University Press, 1978).

42. Ibid., 142. Also see Odin W. Anderson, *Blue Cross Since 1929: Accountability and the Public Trust* (Cambridge, Mass.: Ballinger, 1975), 18.
43. Numbers, "Third Party," 145.
44. Ibid., 147.
45. H. E. Frech and Paul B. Ginsburg, "Competition Among Health Insurers, Revisited," *Journal of Health Politics, Policy and Law* 13 (1988): 279–91. See also Frech and Ginsburg, "Competition Among Health Insurers," in Warren Greenberg, ed., *Competition in the Health Sector: Past, Present, and Future* (Germantown, Md.: Aspen Systems, 1978), and Banks McDowell, *Deregulation and Competition in the Insurance Industry* (New York: Quorum Books, 1989).
46. Samuels, "Documenting Modern Chemistry," 18.
47. The case of E. I. du Pont de Nemours & Co., although not falling into the health industries, provides an example of this type of practice. See David A. Hounshell, "Interpreting the History of Industrial Research and Development: The Case of E. I. du Pont de Nemours & Co.," *Proceedings of the American Philosophical Society* 134 (1990): 387–407. Such a policy at DuPont, according to Hounshell was "designed ostensibly to protect the company" but "comes at an extraordinary high cost: corporate amnesia." [405]
48. See Helen L. Davidson, "The Indispensability of Business Archives," *American Archivist* 30 (1967): 593–97, which is based on her experience at the Eli Lilly and Company Archives, and Davidson, "Selling Management on Business Archives," *ARMA Quarterly* 33 (1969): 15–19, which discusses the types of records to preserve for a firm involved in functions comparable to those discussed in this chapter. An even older report, also based on the Eli Lilly and Company Archives, is Irene M. Strieby, "All the King's Horses . . . ," *Special Libraries* 50 (1959): 425–34. Another argument in favor of businesses maintaining their own archives is John Teresko, "Should You Keep An Archives?" *Industry Week* 188, 15 March 1976, 36–39.
49. Swann, *Scientists and Industry*, 8.
50. The 1988 edition of the National Historical Publications and Records Commission's *Directory of Archives and Manuscript Repositories in the United States* includes only two pharmaceutical entries (Abbott Laboratories and E. R. Squibb & Sons). The health insurance industry has only one entry, that for Blue Cross of California.
51. Some of the companies included are Adac Laboratories, Circadian, Cooper Biomedical, Rasor Associates, and Sierra Scientific.

SELECT ANNOTATED BIBLIOGRAPHY

No single comprehensive study exists for the broad field of health industries, but many examinations of health care in the late twentieth century include discussions of this important segment of the U.S. health care system. One useful source is Joseph A. Califano, Jr., *America's Health Care Revolution: Who*

Lives? Who Dies? Who Pays? (New York: Random House, 1986). Also of use are Stanley Wohl, *The Medical Industrial Complex* (New York: Harmony Books, 1984) and Barbara Ehrenreich and John Ehrenreich, *The American Health Empire: Power, Profits, and Politics* (New York: Random House, 1970). A number of general studies of the pharmaceutical industry are of note. Jonathan Liebenau in *Medical Science and Medical Industry: The Formation of the American Pharmaceutical Industry* (Baltimore: Johns Hopkins University Press, 1987) provides an overview of the development of the industry up to the 1930s with a focus on Philadelphia firms. A work edited by Cotton M. Lindsay, *The Pharmaceutical Industry: Economics, Performance, and Government Regulation* (New York: John Wiley & Sons, 1978), includes several essays on various aspects of the industry. Another essay, "The Pharmaceutical Industry," by Walter S. Measday, in Walter Adams, ed., *The Structure of American Industry*, ed. 5 (New York: Macmillan, 1977), is still of value. A general reference source on the industry is D. J. De Rezno, *Pharmaceutical Manufacturers in the United States.* For an international focus on the industry, see Robert Ballance, Janos Pogany, and Helmut Forstner, *The World's Pharmaceutical Industry: An International Perspective On Innovation, Competition, and Policy* (Brookfield, Vt.: Edward Elgar, 1992).
The medical supplies and equipment industry is less well represented in published works. R. D. Peterson and C. R. MacPhee, *Economic Organization in Equipment and Supply* (Lexington, Mass.: Lexington Books, 1973), is an older treatment of the broad area of this industry. Various government reports on this industry are of more value, including *Federal Policies and the Medical Device Industry* (Washington, D.C.: U.S. Congress, Office of Technology Assessment, 1984). Studies of specific products are available, such as Manuel Trajtenberg, *Economic Analysis of Product Innovation: The Case of CT Scanners* (Cambridge: Harvard University Press, 1990).
For a general overview of the medical publishing industry, see Judith S. Duke, *The Technical, Scientific, and Medical Publishing Market* (White Plains, N.Y.: Knowledge Industry Publications, 1985).
The health insurance industry is perhaps the most widely written about health care industry. Almost any daily newspaper or weekly magazine contains some item on this industry. The standard reference book on health insurance statistics is the annually published *Source Book of Health Insurance Data* (Washington, D.C.: Health Insurance Association of America). Economic aspects of the industry are discussed in Banks McDowell, *Deregulation and Competition in the Insurance Industry* (New York: Quorum Books, 1989). Ronald L. Numbers, *Almost Persuaded: American Physicians and Compulsory Health Insurance, 1912–1920* (Baltimore: Johns Hopkins University Press, 1978) provides historical background to the issue of health insurance in the United States.
A work focusing on the archival aspects of business records, including pharmaceutical companies, is Bruce Bruemmer and Sheldon Hochheiser, *The High-Technology Company: A Historical Research and Archival Guide* (Minneapolis: Charles Babbage Institute, Center for the History of Information Processing, University of Minnesota, 1989).

CHAPTER 8

Documentation Planning and Case Study

JOAN D. KRIZACK

Documentation planning is strategic planning for archives. It is an active process that defines, within an institution or organization, which functions and programs or activities will be documented and to what extent. It also defines the purpose or purposes for which records will be collected: institutional operations,[1] historical research, or, in the case of certain health care institutions, biomedical research. Documentation planning specifies the goals of documentation and outlines methods of attaining the goals. The product of documentation planning is a plan that is more specific than a traditional collecting policy. Grounded in institutional, interinstitutional, and system analyses, the plan identifies specific record series for preservation. Documentation plans are not static; they should be revised regularly to reflect changes in the institution and the larger system of which it is part.[2]

Documentation planning is accomplished in two stages: analysis and selection. The first stage consists of three layers of analysis: (1) an institutional analysis, (2) a comparison of the institution with others of the same type (regionally and nationally),[3] and (3) an analysis of the relationship of the institution to its broader context, in this case the U.S. health care system. The selection stage consists of making decisions at three levels: (1) the function/activity level,[4] (2) the department or subdivision level, and (3) the record series level.

The order in which the first two levels are addressed depends on whether the function is the administration function or a function of a specific type of institution. For example, a hospital's administration function may be broken down into activities (i.e., governance, external rela-

207

tions, fiscal management, operations management, facilities management, and human resources management). Then the archivist identifies the departments and records series that document these activities. All of the remaining functions (i.e., patient care, health promotion, education, and research), however, are documented in each of the medical and ancillary departments. For these functions, the first level of decision-making is the department or subdivision level, the second level is the function level, and the third level is the record series level.

STAGE ONE: ANALYSIS

INSTITUTIONAL ANALYSIS

The basis of documentation planning is an analysis of the institution, its relation to other institutions or organizations of the same type, and its place in the larger environment in which it operates. These internal and external analyses require some time and effort, but they provide a strong foundation for formulating effective documentation plans and performing other archival activities, such as processing and reference.

Institutional analysis consists of five elements:

1. Understanding the institution's mission and defining its functions;
2. Determining whether the institution is freestanding or part of a larger organization (i.e., determining who owns and controls the institution);
3. Understanding how the institution interacts with other institutions, both public and private;
4. Becoming familiar with the institution's history and culture; and
5. Understanding institutional constraints.

Understanding the institution's mission and defining its functions involve identifying the institution's purpose and the broad categories of activities in which it engages. Here it is important to compare the institution's functions with the functions of the U.S. health care system as a whole (see Table 1–1), to identify any functions of the institution that are not health care system functions, and to understand each function's relative importance. A good sense of the institution's mission and functions should emerge from reading its mission statement, bylaws, and recent annual reports. It may also be necessary to peruse management literature related to the type of institution you are documenting to define appropriate functions. This functional analysis is vital to the documentation planning process because it provides a broad overview of the institution and because it is the first and most general level at which documentation decisions are made.

The second element of the institutional analysis is determining whether the institution is freestanding or part of a larger organization or corporation. This is particularly important because it affects where relevant records are likely to be found and who is responsible for their preservation. If the institution is part of a larger body, the archivist must understand its relation and the relation of other subordinate entities to the parent body. This information is necessary if archivists are to have a more complete picture of their own institutions and to determine where, outside of the home institution, significant documentation is likely to reside. Some archivists responsible for institutional records will, of course, be working for the larger organization or corporation. If this is the case, they still need to be concerned about preserving selected records of the subordinate institutions.

Identifying other institutions, public and private, with which your institution interacts and understanding the nature of the interaction is the third element of the institutional analysis. In today's complex society, institutions and organizations are linked to one another through cooperative agreements, funding arrangements, and governmental regulation. These interconnections, which are becoming more frequent and complex in the face of national health care reform, affect the types of record produced, their uniqueness, and their location. By exploring these interinstitutional relationships, archivists may find they need not preserve certain record series because those series are being preserved by another institution. Carrying this idea further, archivists may use the information gleaned from the analysis to initiate cooperative collecting agreements.

The fourth element of the institutional analysis is becoming familiar with the institution's history and culture. Understanding the institution's history enables the archivist to determine whether its functions and their relative importance have changed over time and provides a basis for comparison with other institutions of the same type, which is the next step in the analysis stage of documentation planning. This element of institutional analysis is easily accomplished if a historical volume or a series of historical essays has been written. Otherwise, basic information on the institution's founding, its development, and significant events in its past may be gathered from in-house publications such as annual reports and newsletters, local histories, and other sources.

Institutional culture may be defined as the values, beliefs, and assumptions of an institution. Institutional culture is not necessarily apparent from the records that institutions generate, yet a grasp of the culture is essential to a well-crafted documentation plan. Archivists can begin to understand their institutions' values, beliefs, and assumptions by discussing with appropriate administrators both the formal and the informal channels through which policy is formulated and information is communicated, by acquiring an understanding of how the institution perceives itself and treats its employees, and by learning about the institution's physical environment, employee activities (such as sports competitions and Christmas parties), rituals (service awards), and symbols (logo or seal).[5]

Understanding institutional constraints is the final element of the institutional analysis. Whether the institution is financially sound and has adequate personnel and space is obviously important, because these factors will directly affect the resources available for a records program and therefore the program's scale. If a hospital, for example, is located in the middle of a city where space is costly and there is little room for expansion, the archives program will likely not be assigned adequate on-site storage space. The financial soundness of an institution may be determined by consulting recent annual profit/loss statements (often published in institutional annual reports) or by talking with the institution's chief financial officer. The head of human resources and the institution's facilities planner will be able to provide the information on personnel and space resources.

COMPARISON WITH OTHER INSTITUTIONS OF THE SAME TYPE

The second step in the analysis stage of documentation planning applies the institutional analysis to a broader level, using it to compare a specific institution with other institutions of the same type regionally and nationally. Because such a comparison exposes the usual and unusual aspects of an institution, it is invaluable in formulating the institution's documentation plan. The comparison should be made in terms of the institution's mission, functions, range of activity, size, and significant "first" or "only" accomplishments. Reading institutional histories, if available, and statistical compilations (for example, the American Hospital Association's annual report of hospital statistics) is useful for making interinstitutional comparisons. The lists of institutional types presented in Chapters 2 through 7 may be used to compare health care institutions of various types with their peers. Archivists may also wish to consult their institution's public affairs department, which will be attuned to the special qualities of the institution; however, archivists should keep in mind that this department's mission is to portray the institution in the best light possible.

RELATION TO THE U.S. HEALTH CARE SYSTEM

Broadening the analysis even further, archivists should acquire a general understanding of the U.S. health care system and how their type of institution or organization fits into it. This final layer of analysis, called field analysis, provides the perspective necessary for archivists to place their institutions in a societal context.

An understanding of these three layers of context—institutional, peer, and systemwide (in other words, understanding the institution, its place among similar institutions, and its relationship to the health care system as a whole)—provides a solid foundation on which to build a documentation plan.

STAGE TWO: SELECTION

Once the three layers of analysis have been completed, the documentation plan may be drafted. This is accomplished in four steps:

1. defining the core record series,
2. conducting a retrospective analysis of existing historical materials,
3. conducting departmental studies, and
4. identifying significant record series for archival preservation.

Core record series are the basic series around which archivists should shape their collections.[6] As the foundation of archival collections, core record series are the minimum documentation that should be preserved to document broadly the functions and activities of an institution. Defining the core record series entails first subdividing the institutional administration function into categories of activities. For example, a hospital's administration function, and probably the administrative function of other types of institution as well, might be subdivided into the following categories of activities: governance, external relations, fiscal management, operations management (line activities), facilities management, and human resource management. The administration function is emphasized at this point because by documenting it, an archivist can gain a general overview of the institution and all its functions.

Next, the administrative departments and offices that have significant responsibilities for these activities are listed, along with the important record series that they generate.[7] Archivists should consult the most recent organizational chart, institutional telephone directory, and departmental and institutional annual reports, for example, to be sure they have not overlooked any significant organizational units. It is likely that some organizational units, such as purchasing, will not produce any core records series; if this is the case, they will not appear on the core list. It is important for archivists to begin formulating the list theoretically, but also to work from the reality of what record series are actually created. Although virtually every institution creates annual reports, which are important sources of information and should be part of the core record series, other significant record series may be less obvious.

Some core record series may document more than one function, but they should be listed only under their primary function and the office where the (or an) original is found to avoid confusion and repetition. When the listing of core record series is complete, it should contain only those record series that are necessary to document a function or activity at a general level. (See Table 8–1 for the core record series of Children's Hospital, Boston.)

If the institution already has an archival program in existence or has a cache of historical materials, the archivist needs to conduct a retrospective analysis of existing historical collections to determine generally how well the collections document the institution's functions. Depending on the extent of the records and the complexity of the institution, the archivist may decide to conduct a more specific collection analysis based on the activities and projects that support the institution's functions. Such an analysis is performed by examining all collections and deciding which functions (and then possibly which activities or projects) the collections document, and how well they document the functions over what period of time.[8] The results of this analysis will be more impressionistic than scientific, but they will enable the archivist to assess the collection's strengths and weaknesses, which will be useful information when the documentation plan is written. This information may also lead the archivist to try to locate care record series that are incomplete or missing.

If the institution has no existing archival program, then the archivist should determine whether noncurrent records are stored in a central location. At this point the institution's records manager should be consulted. The purpose of reviewing these noncurrent record series is to determine how well they document the institution's functions, activities, or projects and which of them should be preserved in the archives. This analysis should also include an assessment of significant record series that have been lost or destroyed (if they can be identified) and the functions they would have documented. Again, this analysis will inform the documentation plan.

The next step in the selection process involves studying the institution's medical departments and other nonadministrative units. The functions other than institutional administration (i.e., patient care, health

TABLE 8–1   Children's Hospital's core records series

All Functions (function level)
All departments, and other organization units (organizational unit level)
  Annual reports of the department/unit (record series level)
  Departmental committee minutes
  Departmental organization charts
  Departmental policy and procedure manuals
  Departmental publications (e.g., newsletters, brochures, updates)
  Photographs, films, slides, etc., of department staff, interiors, and events

Institutional Administration (function level)
External Relations (activity level)
  CEO's office (organizational unit level)
    Correspondence file (record series level)
  Department of Development and Public Affairs
    Official institution publications (*The News, Children's Today, Children's World, Inside Children's, Pediatric Views*)
    Photograph/slide files
    Press releases
    Promotional videotapes of Children's Hospital
  Governmental and Community Relations Office
    Correspondence file
Fiscal Management
  Vice President for Finance's office
    Annual profit/loss statements
    Audited financial reports (institutional)
Operations Management
  Research Administration
    Investigator profiles (annual compilation of institutional research activity)
    Committee minutes (Enders Faculty Council Steering, Awards, Education, Facilities, Research Computing, and Technology Transfer)
  Vice President of Medical Affairs' Office
    Medical staff bylaws
    Medical staff correspondence file
    Medical staff directories
    Minutes of medical staff standing committees (Cardiopulmonary Resuscitation Committee, Clinical Investigation, Credentials, Disaster Control, Ethics Advisory, Infection Control, Medical Records, Medical Staff Executive, Nutrition Advisory, Oncology, Pharmacy, Quality Improvement, Radiation Safety, Senior Appointments, Special Care Units [Multidisciplinary Intensive Care Unit, Cardiac ICU and Newborn ICU], Tissue, and Transfusion)
    Rules and regulations of the medical staff
  Vice President for Operations' Office
    Resident Handbooks
Facilities Management
  CEO's Office
    Property deeds

(continued)

TABLE 8–1   Children's Hospital's core records series   *(continued)*

Facilities Management *(continued)*
  Engineering office
    Blueprints for building(s)
  Facility Planning office
    Planning reports
    Photographs/slides of buildings
    Correspondence file
  Vice President for Operations
    Correspondence file

Human Resource Management
  CEO's office
    Professional staff correspondence
  Communications
    Children's Hospital telephone directories
  Human Resources
    Employee handbook
    Hospital policy and procedure manuals

Governance
  CEO's office
    Annual or periodic reports of CEO
    Articles of incorporation
    Charter
    Constitution and bylaws
    Minutes of medical center/hospital standing committees (Audit, Develop-
      ment, Executive, Facility Planning, Finance, Investment, and Patient Care
      Assessment)
    Organizational charts

Patient Care
Admitting, Emergency Services, and Operating Room
  patient logs (currently online)

Development and Public Affairs office
  Directory of Medical Staff and Ambulatory Programs

Medical Records Department
  Disease index (online after 1979)
  Patient records index (online after 1979)

Department of Laboratory Medicine
  Laboratory handbooks

Health Promotion
Health Information Department
  Occasional publications

Education
Human Resources
  Training Handbook

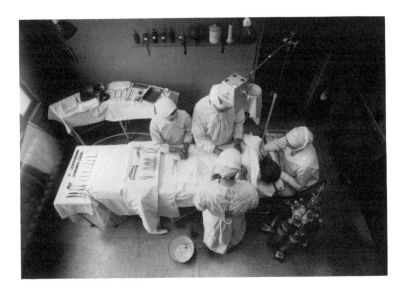

FIGURE 8–1   Operating room in Children's Hospital, Boston, 1932.   *Source:* Children's Hospital Archives

promotion, education, and biomedical research) are emphasized from this point forward. The selection process now changes from that used to identify the core record series: the organizational units become the first level of selection, after which come the function/activity level and then the record series level. This process is appropriate because in most of the U.S. health care system's institutions the patient care, health promotion, education, and biomedical research activities are inextricably linked at the departmental level. The first step is to list the medical and other nonadministrative departments. These units may be subdivided as necessary. For example, at Children's Hospital some of the medical departments are subdivided into divisions and subdivisions. (See Table 8–2.) Then the archivist conducts a study of each organizational unit, talking with the unit's head or another designated representative and the individuals responsible for managing the unit's records to better understand how it is organized and what it does. Through this process the archivist gathers background information and determines what core record series the department generates (e.g., departmental annual reports, minutes of departmental committees, photographs and other audiovisual materials, departmental newsletters or other publications, departmental policy and

TABLE 8–2　Departments or services engaging in patient care, health promotion, biomedical research, and educational activities

Medical Departments

Anesthesia

Cardiology and Cardiovascular Surgery

Dentistry

Medicine
　Adolescent and Young Adult Medicine
　Emergency Medicine
　Endocrinology
　Gastroenterology and Nutrition (one program)
　　Clinical Gastroenterology and Nutrition
　General Pediatrics (eleven programs)
　　Child Development Unit
　　Clinical Pediatrics Program
　　Community and Support Services
　　Comprehensive Child Health
　　Developmental Evaluation Center
　　Family Development Program
　　Martha Eliot Health Center
　　Medical Diagnostic Programs
　　Pediatric Group Associates
　　Pharmacology-Toxicology Program
　　Services to Handicapped Children
　Genetics (one program)
　　Clinical Genetics
　Hematology and Oncology
　Immunology (four programs)
　　Allergy
　　Dermatology
　　Clinical Immunology
　　Rheumatology
　Infectious Diseases
　Nephrology
　Newborn Medicine
　Pulmonary Medicine (one program)
　　Cystic Fibrosis Research Laboratories
　Inpatient Services (eight programs)
　　Blackfan Service (school-aged children)
　　Bone Marrow Transplantation Service
　　Clinical Research Center Service
　　Janeway Service (adolescents)
　　Medical Intensive Care Service
　　Neonatal Intensive Care Service

(continued)

TABLE 8–2 Departments or services engaging in patient care, health promotion, biomedical research, and educational activities *(continued)*

Inpatient Services (eight programs) *(continued)*
 Oncology Service
 Rotch Service (infants and toddlers)
Neurology
Neurosurgery
Ophthalmology
Orthopaedic Surgery
 Sports Medicine
Otolaryngology and Communication Disorders
 Communication Enhancement Center
Pathology
Psychiatry
 Psychology
Radiation Therapy
Radiology
 Nuclear Medicine
Surgery
 Gynecology
 Plastic Surgery
 Urology

Other Nonadministrative Departments/Units
Department of Laboratory Medicine
Information Service
Nursing
Nutrition and Food Service
Pastoral Care
Patient Activities
Pharmacy
Physical Therapy
Quality Improvement
Respiratory Therapy
Social Work
Utilization Review
Volunteers

---

procedure manuals). The archivist then identifies for preservation any additional record series that best document the department.[9]

It is possible to decide not to document a particular division or subdivision beyond the information contained in department-level records. If, however, a division or subdivision is identified for further documentation, it is necessary for the archivist to meet with the division head to identify record series for preservation. I found medical department chiefs helpful in identifying those divisions and subdivisions significant enough to be documented beyond the general level of information provided by records at the department level.

The selection process will assuredly not progress as smoothly as suggested here. There may be times when records must be appraised before the documentation plan has been completed because a department is moving or an individual is retiring or has died, and there may be times when a deparment head refuses to cooperate in the documentation planning process. Although documentation plans are formulated from the top down, the planning process also involves simultaneously working at the unit level from the record series up. There is no specific formula that can be used, but the archivist's ability to move from conceptualization to archival reality and back again is essential to crafting a good plan.

At this point, if the institution is limiting its collecting scope to archival records, the documentation plan is complete. If, however, the institution wishes to acquire manuscript materials (papers of individuals and records of outside organizations) or artifacts to complement its archival records, then the documentation plan should conclude with detailed selection criteria for manuscripts and artifacts. These criteria are part of a traditional collecting policy.

DOCUMENTATION PLANNING: PRACTICAL ASPECTS

The first part of this chapter defined a documentation plan and described the components of the planning process: background analysis and selection. The remainder of this chapter describes the practical aspects of documentation planning and provides an example of a portion of a documentation plan, that formulated for Children's Hospital, Boston.

ADMINISTRATIVE FOUNDATION

Building institutional support at various levels is critical to successful documentation planning. After the archivist enlists the support of her or his immediate supervisor, the next step is to gain the active support of the institution's chief executive officer (CEO) for the program. In fact, it is helpful if the archivist sends out a letter, over the CEO's signature, to all departments explaining the documentation planning project and requesting their cooperation. To gain CEO support, however, it may first be necessary to have the support of other administrators, such as vice presidents, legal counsel, department heads, and laboratory directors. Realistically, in some institutions it may not be possible to obtain the support of key administrators. In that case, gather whatever support you can while you keep trying to win the support of the other institutional leaders. The worst case is that you may have to wait for top-level support until the administration changes.

ARCHIVES COMMITTEE

While the archivist is securing the authority to carry out the documentation planning project, the archives committee is assembled. The committee should consist of records creators, users, and preservers: the archivist, the records manager (who may be the same individual as the archivist), the librarian, key administrators from each functional area, historians of medicine or other historical researchers interested in topics documented by the institution's records, a representative from the institution's legal department, and a trustee or overseer. If the CEO or executive vice president can be enlisted to serve on the committee, so much the better. Others may be added to the team as appropriate. In the case of a hospital that engages in biomedical research, for example, a physician, the medical records specialist, and a biomedical researcher should be recruited to serve on the committee. Although the archivist will effectively chair the committee, it is important that another committee member be the nominal chair. Someone with greater institutional influence will usually be more effective in accomplishing the committee's goals. In the hospital setting, a senior staff physician or vice president is an appropriate archives committee chair.

DOCUMENTATION PLAN ARTICULATION

The heart of the documentation planning process is writing the documentation plan. As mentioned earlier, the plan specifies what will be documented within each department and identifies specific record series that will be preserved in the archives. Once information on existing historical collections and/or noncurrent record series has been accumulated, the archivist engages in additional analytical work, classifying the medical and other nonadministrative departments and their subunits. The next steps are to understand departmental functions and activities, and finally to identify the record series that document their functions.

After selected record series have been designated to come to the archives, the documentation plan is complete. For institutions or organizations founded before the post–World War II "information explosion" the archives committee may wish to select a date before which all or virtually all records will be kept. It should be emphasized that the archivist begins formulating the documentation plan theoretically, but as the records are reviewed, the plan will be revised as necessary to reflect the reality of what records are actually generated. Annual notices should be sent to organizational units to remind them of their agreement to send specified material to the archives, and completed plans should be reviewed and updated every few years or when departments are merged or disbanded.

The archives committee should also decide whether the papers of individuals, the records of other organizations, and artifacts should be sought to complement the archival collection. If manuscript material and artifacts are to be collected, the documentation plan should specify which individuals and/or types of organization should be solicited, taking into consideration strengths and weaknesses of the archival collections. Members of the archives committee will undoubtedly be helpful in identifying individuals whose papers should be preserved.

In the hospital settings in which there is no records management program, I have found it useful to have the archives program part of the development and public affairs department rather than a function of the hospital library. This is because development and public affairs staff members have a broad understanding of the institution and how it operates. They have their fingers on the pulse of the institution, understand individual personalities, and can provide valuable advice on how to accomplish documentation planning goals. There is, however, the danger that the development and public affairs staff will view the archives solely in terms of fund-raising and public relations activities.

CASE STUDY: CHILDREN'S HOSPITAL, BOSTON
INSTITUTIONAL ANALYSIS

Element 1: Mission and Functions   The original mission of Children's Hospital, as stated by the Board of Managers in 1869, was threefold: "The medical and surgical treatment of the diseases of children. The attainment and diffusion of knowledge regarding the diseases incident to childhood.

The training of young women in the duties of nursing."[10] The hospital's current bylaws expand and clarify this mission:

> The mission of Children's Hospital is to provide excellent health care to children and, in support of this mission, to be the leading source of research and discovery, seeking new approaches to the prevention, diagnosis and treatment of childhood diseases as well as to educate the next generation of leaders in child health.

In the nearly 125 years since the mission was first articulated, the institution's basic functions of patient care, biomedical research, and education have remained the same. Patient care is now clearly stated as the primary function, health promotion and community outreach activities play a prominent role in the institution, and although the school of nursing closed in 1978, the hospital still considers the education of nurses, physicians, technicians, and others as one of its primary functions. Children's Hospital is therefore involved in four of the six functions of the U.S. health care system. Additionally, like all institutions, Children's Hospital engages in institutional administration, a function that includes a range of activities necessary to keep the institution running: governance, external relations, fiscal management, operations management, facilities management, and human resource management. These activities tend to be similar in institutions of all types.

As the current mission statement makes clear, the primary function of Children's Hospital is patient care. The hospital is a tertiary care facility and provides the full range of services from standard, noncritical care through specialized care and experimental treatment of infants, children, and adolescents with extremely complex and virtually unique medical conditions. The hospital is organized into fourteen clinical departments with nineteen divisions that are further subdivided into twenty-seven programs. Children's Hospital also offers more than 100 outpatient programs. Health promotion is closely allied to its patient care activities. Although not explicitly stated in its mission statement, the Children's Hospital bylaws (1989) emphasize health promotion through prevention. The bylaws state that among its purposes are "to instruct, supervise, and train [health care professionals] in the care, treatment, and prevention of diseases . . . and to determine new and improved methods for the treatment and prevention of diseases, and to disseminate information about such matters."

Children's Hospital is the largest pediatric research facility in the world and stands fourth among all independent hospitals in research funding from the National Institutes of Health.[11] The John F. Enders Pediatric Research Laboratories at Children's Hospital house more than

500 researchers, and in 1992 the hospital was awarded $34 million for research ($23 million from federal sources, $4 million from the Howard Hughes Medical Institute, $3 million from industry, $3 million from foundations, and the remainder from other sources, including the Commonwealth of Massachusetts). From fiscal years 1987 through 1992, research funding continued to grow, despite the increasing scarcity of and competition for research dollars, especially from the federal government.

Children's Hospital is the primary Harvard Medical School teaching hospital for pediatrics, but its educational activities are not limited to training physicians. In addition to internships, residencies, and postgraduate programs for physicians, several departments also offer advanced training programs for doctoral and postdoctoral students in the medical sciences. The departments of Anesthesia, Cardiology and Cardiovascular Surgery, and Medicine, for example, organize complete courses taught by staff members. In other departments, including Orthopaedics and Neurosurgery, staff members present pediatric aspects within general courses on their specialties. The hospital plays an important role in educating pediatric nurse clinicians. The Department of Nursing is affiliated with twenty academic institutions throughout the United States and provides education at the baccalaureate, master's, and doctoral levels.

Children's Hospital also offers, among other programs, internships in dietetics, social service, pastoral care, and clinical psychology; residencies in pharmacy and hospital administration; formal on-the-job training programs for electrocardiograph technicians, housekeeping aides, respiratory therapy technicians, and surgical technicians; affiliated programs in physical therapy with Boston University, Simmons College, and Northeastern University, and in radiologic technology with Northeastern; informal on-the-job training for laboratory technicians, unit secretaries, industrial engineers, and autopsy attendants; and continuing education to meet the recertification criteria of many health professions. Nearly every administrative and medical department at Children's Hospital is involved in providing educational experiences for students who will be future health care professionals.

Element 2: Institutional Control   Children's Hospital is considered a freestanding institution by the National Association of Children's Hospitals and Related Institutions (NACHRI), although it is formally part of a holding company, Children's Medical Center. Children's Medical Center comprises Children's Hospital, the Children's National Research Institute (which is currently inactive, but may be activated in the future to provide organizational structure for research activities conducted by the Hospital),

Children's Extended Care Center (Groton, Massachusetts), Fenmore Realty Corporation (a nonprofit corporation formed to acquire income-producing real estate), Longwood Associates, Inc. (a for-profit subsidiary that manages the Medical Center's real estate development), and the Longwood Corporation (a nonprofit corporation owning real property for the benefit of its nonprofit parent). The hospital runs two satellites: the Martha Eliot Health Center (Jamaica Plain, a suburb of Boston), a neighborhood clinic, and the Children's Hospital Specialty Care Center (Lexington, Massachusetts), an outpatient referral facility. The Children's Hospital League, a subsidiary of the hospital, is a nonprofit corporation operated by volunteers; it plans and conducts various fund-raising events for the hospital's benefit.

The Children's Medical Center is governed by a board of fifteen trustees that is identical to the hospital's board. The standing committees of the Children's Medical Center are the Audit Committee, Development Committee, Executive Committee, Facility Planning Committee, Finance Committee, Investment Committee, and Patient Care Assessment Committee. (It should be noted that the standing committees of all institutions or organizations change with regularity.)

Element 3: Interactions with Other Institutions   Children's Hospital is linked to many other institutions in carrying out activities related to patient care. As examples, it has joint programs with Beth Israel Hospital, Brigham and Women's Hospital, Dana-Farber Cancer Institute, Judge Baker Children's Center, Massachusetts General Hospital, and the New England Deaconess Hospital. In biomedical research it has joint programs with Aga Khan University in Karachi, Pakistan; Harvard University's Department of Biochemistry and Molecular Biology; the Massachusetts Institute of Technology National Magnet Laboratory; the Whitehead Institute in Cambridge, Massachusetts; and Digital Equipment Corporation. In research funding joint programs include those with the National Institutes of Health, the Howard Hughes Medical Institute, the American Health Association, and the Commonwealth of Massachusetts, among others. In education it shares programs with Harvard Medical School (twenty-five courses were listed in the 1991–1992 catalogue that third- and fourth-year medical students could take at Children's Hospital), Boston English High School, Bunker Hill Community College, Simmons College, and most Boston teaching hospitals. Joint programs in administration include those with the Massachusetts Hospital Association, NACHRI, and the Medical Area Service Corporation, which provides transportation, purchasing, and other services to institutions in the Longwood Medical Area, and with accreditation and regulatory organizations such as the Joint Commission on Accreditation of Healthcare Organizations and the Occupational Safety and Health Administration.

Because it is located in the Longwood Medical Area, which is home to six health care delivery facilities,[12] Harvard Medical School, Harvard School of Public Health, Harvard School of Dental Medicine, Harvard's Francis A. Countway Library of Medicine, the Forsyth Dental Center School for Dental Hygienists, and the Massachusetts College of Pharmacy and Allied Health Sciences, every conceivable kind of affiliation, formal or informal, has developed between Children's Hospital and the surrounding medical community over the years. Much of this interaction had been intended to improve care for patients, but with increased frequency joint programs are coming into existence for education at all levels, and for biomedical research. Because Children's interinstitutional connections are extensive and complex and represent all four of the institution's functions, they will be investigated in more detail at the organizational unit level.

Element 4: History and Culture   Children's Hospital was chartered by the legislature of the Commonwealth of Massachusetts in 1869. Its history, from the hospital's founding through the early 1980s, has been recorded in two books and a pamphlet. From my reading of these historical works and serial publications of the Development and Public Affairs Department, certain facts that helped to shape the documentation plan began to emerge. For example:

• The nation's first pediatric radiology department was established at Children's Hospital in 1900.
• In 1903 the informal ties to Harvard Medical School were formalized; hospital chiefs of service from this time on hold positions at Harvard.
• In 1914 Children's Hospital was one of the first U.S. hospitals of any type to create an independent physical therapy department.
• In 1938 Dr. Robert Gross performed the world's first successful surgical procedure to correct a cardiovascular defect, laying the foundation for modern cardiac surgery.
• In 1947 Children's Hospital made the transition to Children's Medical Center, becoming the first pediatric medical center in the country.

From the perspective of documentation planning, one of the most important points that becomes clear is that the health care delivery, biomedical research, and education functions are closely integrated. Patient care has always been the primary function of Children's; biomedical research, mentioned prominently in the original mission statement of the hospital, was the second function, with education following closely. It is important to note that when research at Children's Hospital came into its own in the early 1920s it did so within the existing departmental structure, rather than as a separate department or organization devoted to biomedical research. The implications for documentation planning are clear: because the health care delivery, biomedical research, and education functions are integrated, it is expedient to plan to document these functions within selected hospital departments or divisions instead of as isolated functions. At the same time, it is important to have an overview of the functions and to think functionally when devising the documentation plan. The exception is the institutional administration function which operates separately from the other functions and is therefore documented independently.

From the vantage point of an employee, Children's Hospital's institutional culture is readily apparent. The institution has a strong sense of tradition and is proud of its history. For example, an annual lecture on the history of the institution has been given for many years and is well-attended. Employees at all levels are conscious of Children's leadership role in pediatric medicine and are proud of being part of what they consider a special enterprise. The hospital is compassionate both to its employees, who are valued, and to its patients, who receive a remarkably high level of care. On occasion, for example, Children's Hospital has found funding to pay transportation costs to Boston for a dying child's grandparents. The culture of Children's Hospital is also permeated with ambition; individuals are personally ambitious, and the institution is ambitious for children, believing that with hard work all barriers to pediatric health can be overcome.

The culture of Children's Hospital may be summed up in the words of George H. Kidder, chairman of the Children's Hospital Board of Trustees: "Children's is about people, and being mindful of the human side of this place is the key to guiding it into the future. Building solid, supportive, and trusting relationships is the way to ensure that this hospital fulfills its mission of providing the finest care to children."[13] Supporting this tradition of compassion and trust is Children's logo—a nurse closely holding a child.

Element 5: Institutional Constraints   The hospital's operating budget for fiscal year 1992 was $255.3 million, and it ended the year with a favorable balance of $24.5 million. The hospital gained $7.7 million from patient care operations and $28 million from favorable prior year adjustments. However, $11.2 million was used to refinance debt.

Viewed over a seven-year period (FY 1986–1992), the institution's financial situation is strong. Audited surpluses were recorded for the entire period, ranging from a low of $0.2 million in 1989 to a high of $24.5 million in 1992. Also, after experiencing four years (1986–1989) of negative cash flow, the hospital reported significant positive cash flow in FY 1990–1992. The period of negative cash flow is accounted for by the construction costs for two buildings that were added to improve facilities for in-patient care and research.

It should also be noted that the Commonwealth of Massachusetts adopted new hospital finance legislation (Chapter 495) on December 31, 1991. This law deregulates hospital revenues, allowing hospitals to nego-tiate discounts with managed care organizations and insurers. At the same time, the legislation significantly reduced Children's reimbursement from the Commonwealth for bad debts and free care. The long-term implica-tions for Children's Hospital, while not altogether clear, are optimistically viewed by its administration. In addition it is not clear how the Clinton administration's health care reforms, which emphasize competition and managed care, will affect Children's. The hospital is already planning how to change to remain competitive in the new environment.

COMPARISON OF CHILDREN'S HOSPITAL WITH OTHER CHILDREN'S HOSPITALS, NATIONALLY AND REGIONALLY

There are 149 freestanding children's hospitals in the United States and 42 that are part of a larger organization.[14] Of the freestanding institutions, 45 are children's general hospitals comparable to Children's Hospital. In New England there are only 2 other freestanding children's general hospitals: Newington (Connecticut) Children's Hospital and Hasbro Children's Hospital in Providence, Rhode Island. There is one listing for a New England children's hospital that is not freestanding: the Floating Hospital for Infants and Children at New England Medical Center.

These statistics, together with the fact that Children's Hospital is the largest pediatric research facility in the country, clearly indicate that the hospital is close to being a unique institution within New England. (It is also the only freestanding children's hospital in the country to have a full-time professional archivist.)

ANALYSIS OF CHILDREN'S HOSPITAL'S RELATIONSHIP TO THE U.S. HEALTH CARE SYSTEM

This analysis involves reading through Chapter 1, "An Overview of the United States Health Care System," and Chapter 2, "Health Care Delivery

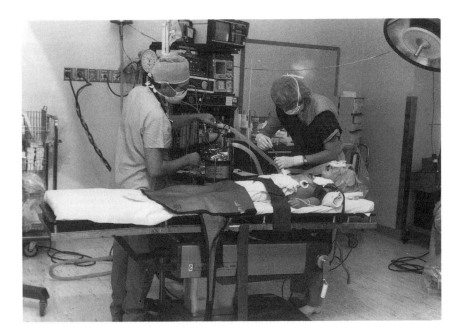

FIGURE 8–2   Dental operating room in Children's Hospital, Boston, 1992.
Source: Development and Public Affairs Office, Children's Hospital

Facilities," to gain a perspective on the U.S. health care system and the role of hospitals within it. These chapters also help point out the types of relationship a hospital might have with other institutions and organizations that are part of the U.S. health care system and indicate some of the changes in the system that can be expected with the advent of health care reform.

STAGE TWO: SELECTION

WHY WILL RECORDS BE COLLECTED?

The Archives Committee decided that archival materials would be collected primarily for institutional operations and historical research purposes. Secondarily, they will be collected for biomedical research purposes.[15] The implication is that research data may not always be maintained in the hospital's archives; however, the archivist will attempt to find an appropriate repository for research data that is not housed in the archives.

The Archives Committee also decided that documenting the medical components of Children's Medical Center (the Hospital and Children's

Specialty Care Center) would take precedence over documenting the real estate components of the Medical Center.

SELECTION: FUNCTION LEVEL

This is the most general level—the level where the selection process begins. Of the five functions of Children's Hospital (patient care, health promotion, biomedical research, education, and institutional administration) the Archives Committee agreed to emphasize the administration and biomedical research functions. Administration will be emphasized because of the institution's virtually unique position in New England, because by documenting administrative activities thoroughly, all of the other functions will be documented generally, and because documenting the administrative function will be helpful in carrying out current hospital administrative activities. Biomedical research will be another focus of the documentation plan because of Children's position as the largest pediatric research facility in the world and because the institution has significant accomplishments in this area. The documentation plan will also focus on health promotion because it is an area of activity that is gaining in importance owing to the federal government's emphasis on cost containment and managed care.

Patient care will be documented by virtue of the fact that Children's Hospital has retained all of its patient records and logs since it opened in 1869. This decision was made before the documentation planning effort began.[16] Patient care is also documented in the multitude of articles written about patients and published in the various official publications originating in the Development and Public Affairs Office and constituting the recommended core documentation. Education is more difficult to document because much of it is done in conjunction with other (usually educational) institutions that have archival programs where the bulk of the documentation resides. The Francis A. Countway Library of Medicine, for example, hold materials documenting aspects of the classroom education of Harvard medical students who received clinical training at Children's. For this reason, the documentation plan will place slightly less emphasis on education.

SELECTION: ORGANIZATIONAL UNIT LEVEL

The first step is to identify the medical and other nonadministrative departments, indicating their divisions, subdivisions, and programs as appropriate. Table 8–2 outlines the territory to be documented. Originally I thought that with the Archives Committee's help I would be able to designate certain departments that would be documented only by the core documentation (i.e., departmental annual reports; minutes of departmental committee meetings; photographs of departmental staff, events, and interiors; departmental policy and procedure manuals; and department publications, such as newsletters and brochures). After talking with the Archives Committee, it became clear to me that this approach would not work at Children's Hospital because everyone thinks that his or her department is important and worthy of being fully documented in the Hospital Archives. Although all medical departments will be documented, not all of the departmental divisions and subdivisions will be documented beyond the level of documentation residing in the department chief's files.

The Anesthesia Department was the first to be studied for documentation possibilities. One reason for this was purely practical—the associate chief of the department was a member of the Archives Committee and sympathetic to the documentation planning process. Other reasons were that the Anesthesia Department was not well documented in existing archival records and that the department is relatively small and not complex, thus providing a good starting point. As a first step, I did background research by rereading the sections of the hospital histories devoted to the anesthesia department and reading through the last five years of departmental annual reports. Then I met with the chief, the associate chief, the clinical director of the Pain Treatment Service (which is one of three department subdivisions that the associate chief recommended be documented more fully), and the department administrator. I used the questions and topics listed in Table 8–3 as the basis of the meeting. (The questions in Table 8–4 may be used as a basis for developing documentation plans for administrative departments.) The documentation plan for the Department of Anesthesia was reviewed by the three physicians and the department administrator who were interviewed. The final report was signed and dated by the department chief and the archivist and distributed to appropriate people within the department.

DEPARTMENT OF ANESTHESIA DOCUMENTATION PLAN
DEPARTMENTAL ORGANIZATION

The department is organized into four divisions and one subdivision, all of which are among the largest such programs in the country:

- cardiac anesthesia
- multidisciplinary intensive care unit (MICU)
- division of respiratory therapy

TABLE 8–3 Checklist of questions and topics for medical departmental analysis

---

1. Is the department organized into divisions/sections?
2. Describe the patient care (inpatient and outpatient) activities of the department.
3. Describe the health promotion activities of the department.
4. Describe the teaching (predoctoral, resident, fellow, technologist, continuing education, etc.) activities of the department.
5. Describe the research (clinical and basic) activities of the department.
6. What are the departmentwide committees?
7. What is unusual about the department?
8. What is most important to document about the department?
9. What record series are needed in documenting this?
10. Describe the electronic records systems in place.
11. Does the department generate:
    a. Annual reports?
    b. Departmental newsletters, patient brochures, information sheets, or other publications?
    c. Photographs or other audiovisual materials?
    d. Committee minutes?
    e. Policy and procedure manuals?
    f. Departmental organization charts?
    g. Records of teaching activities?
    h. Records of research activities?
    i. Patient records other than official medical records?
12. Has a departmental history been written?
13. Are there caches of departmental records that are not being used for current operations? If yes, where are they located?

- operating room
- pain treatment service

The department has several committees: Clinical Competence, Education, Fellowship Selection, Quality Assurance, and Research.

PATIENT CARE

The department is one of the largest pediatric anesthesia departments in the world, and its services are used for every possible type of pediatric

TABLE 8–4 Checklist of questions and topics for administrative department analysis

---

1. Is the department organized into divisions/sections?
2. What are the departmental functions?
3. Does the department operate special programs?
4. What are the departmentwide committees?
5. What is unusual about the department?
6. What is most important to document about the department?
7. What record series are needed to document this?
8. Describe the electronic records systems in place.
9. Does the department generate:
   a. Annual reports?
   b. Departmental newsletters, patient brochures, information sheets, or other publications?
   c. Photographs or other audiovisual materials?
   d. Committee minutes?
   e. Policy and procedure manuals?
   f. Departmental organization charts?
   g. Records of teaching activities?
   h. Records of research activities?
   i. Patient records other than official medical records
10. Has a departmental history been written?
11. Are there caches of departmental records that are not being used for current operations? If yes, where are they located?

---

operation and for many procedures done outside the operating rooms, such as diagnostic radiology and radiation therapy.

TEACHING

The department has what is probably the largest anesthesiology training program in the United States, educating residents and fellows and providing continuing education programs for physicians. Residents from Beth Israel Hospital, Brigham and Women's Hospital, University Hospital, St. Elizabeth's Hospital, Massachusetts General Hospital (MGH), and occasionally others rotate through Children's for two to three months. At any given time, the department has about fifteen residents. Fellows come for between six months and three years to become specialized in pediatric anesthesiology and/or pediatric critical care medicine. The department is involved with two continuing education programs—an anesthesia review course with MGH, and the Harvard Medical School Department of Anesthesia's review course.

RESEARCH

The department engages in a significant amount of research, publishing over 100 papers per year. It participates in the Harvard Anesthesia Center Research Grant (HACRG), which is run out of MGH. The program, which has been funded by NIH for more than 20 years, trains anesthesiologists in research. Participation in the HACRG program may lead to a Ph.D. from Harvard or MIT.

Other research is organized by division, and all faculty are encouraged to engage in research activities. Cardiac Anesthesia engages in clinical studies and conducts basic research in conjunction with the Department of Cardiology and Cardiovascular Surgery; the Multidisciplinary Intensive Care Unit engages in clinical and basic research involving critically ill patients; operating room staff do clinical research; the Pain Treatment Service has its own laboratory and engages in clinical and basic research studies.

PAIN TREATMENT SERVICE

Established in 1986, the Pain Treatment Service is the first multidisciplinary children's pain service in the world. Its primary staff is composed of anesthesiologists, psychologists, nurses, and physical therapists. Annually, 2,000 children (in-patients and outpatients) are treated for postoperative pain and pain associated with cancer. The patient records and shadow patient files of the service are computerized and never purged.

RECORD SERIES IDENTIFIED FOR PRESERVATION IN THE ARCHIVES

All functions:
- Department annual reports (published in "Reports of the Departments"; currently have 1976–1992)
- Department chief's correspondence files

Patient Care:
- Clinical Competence Committee minutes
- Quality Assurance Committee minutes
- Pain Treatment Service brochures

- Pain Treatment Service pain management protocols
- Pain Treatment Service patient handouts (e.g., on pediatric cancer pain)

Education
- Annual syllabi of review courses
- Calendar of daily lectures and seminars (issued monthly)
- Education Committee minutes
- Educational manuals for trainees (produced by each division)
- Fellowship Selection Committee minutes
- Staff, resident, and fellow lists
- Trainee and staff file

Research
- Pain Treatment Service correspondence file
- Research Committee minutes
- Staff bibliography (in department's annual reports)

Health promotion
    The department does not engage in health promotion activities

Other
- Photographs of staff and fellows (taken annually)
- Final budget performance reports
- Main Operating Room
- Anesthesia Laboratory
- Pain Service

DOCUMENTATION PLANNING: A METHODOLOGY FOR SPECIALIZED APPLICATION

The documentation plan for Children's Hospital Anesthesia Department is an application of the documentation planning process to a particular department in a specialized hospital. The plan is not meant to be a plan for all anesthesia departments in all hospitals, but illustrates the documentation planning processes of analysis (institutional, interinstitutional, and field) and selection (at the function/activity, department/program, and record series levels). The process was designed to be translated to other hospital organizational units and to the other institutions and organizations composing the U.S. health care system.

On an even more general level, the documentation planning process can be applied to institutions and organizations outside of the U.S. health care system, such as state or local government institutions, arts organizations, and labor organizations. To develop documentation plans for institutions or organizations that are not part of the U.S. health care system, archivists will first need to develop field analyses, such as this book provides for health care, for the larger systems of which these other institutions and organizations are a part.

NOTES

1. "Institutional" may also be read as "organizational" throughout this chapter.
2. Documentation planning is an intrainstitutional approach to selection; documentation strategy is an interinstitutional approach. See Helen Willa Samuels, "Who Controls the Past?" *American Archivist* 49 (Spring 1986): 109–24. It is my belief that if documentation strategies are possible, they are only so after the institutions involved have formulated documentation plans.
3. In some cases it may also be appropriate to examine the community context. For example, when documenting a hospital in a large urban setting, it is important to compare the hospital to others in and around the city.
4. Functions may be subdivided into subfunctions or activities as the case requires. For example, in this book health care delivery has been divided into patient care and health promotion in an attempt to emphasize health promotion, which otherwise might not be appropriately documented.
5. Cynthia G. Swank, "Organizational Culture and Its Role in the Creation, Survival and Use of Records: A Case Study" (Paper delivered at the Bentley Historical Collections Symposium, July 1990).
6. The idea of core documentation is adapted from the library world's concept of core collection. See, for example, Samuels, "Who Controls the Past?" 113–14.
7. Invoices for office supplies and other "housekeeping" records, for example, are not significant record series for the purpose of documentation planning.
8. See Judith E. Endelman, "Looking Backward to Plan for the Future: Collection Analysis for Manuscript Repositories," *American Archivist* 50 (Summer 1987): 340–53. Endelman's approach could be adapted to an institutional archives.
9. It took me seven or eight hours from start to finish to devise the documentation plan for the Children's Hospital Anesthesia Department.
10. *The Children's Hospital: 1869–1939* (no publisher, n.d.), 9.
11. "Independent" is the operative word. Many hospitals are affiliated with a university, and their research funding is reported as part of the research funding of the parent institution.
12. The six are Beth Israel, Brigham and Women's, Children's, New England Deaconess, Dana-Farber Cancer Institute, and Joslin Diabetes Center.
13. *Children's World: Year in Review 1991*, 5.
14. All statistics in this section are taken from *Listing of Freestanding Children's Hospitals in the United States* compiled by the National Association of Children's Hospitals and Related Institutions (NACHRI). NACHRI's source was the 1991

edition of the *American Hospital Association Guide to the Health Care Field* which
was based on the American Hospital Association's 1990 annual survey.

15. It should be noted that Nancy McCall and Lisa Mix, editors of *Designing
Archival Programs to Advance Knowledge in the Health Fields* (Baltimore: Johns
Hopkins University Press, 1994), recommend that preserving material for
biomedical research purposes be a primary function of health-related
archives; however, Children's Hospital was not ready to commit the
necessary resources.

16. For an excellent discussion of the secondary uses of official patient records
and appraisal considerations for patient records, see Joel D. Howell,
"Preserving Patient Records to Support Health Care Delivery, Teaching, and
Research," in Nancy McCall and Lisa Mix, eds., *Designing Archival Programs to
Advance Knowledge in the Health Fields* (Baltimore: Johns Hopkins University
Press, 1994).

Selected Landmarks in the History of Health Care in the United States

1756	Oldest U.S. hospital, Pennsylvania Hospital (Philadelphia), founded.
1760	First physician licensing statute enacted in New York City.
1765	First medical school in the United States, Medical School of the College of Philadelphia, founded.
1766	First colonial, later state, medical society founded in New Jersey.
1772	New Jersey act regulating medical practice; colonial, later state, board of medical examiners adopted by New Jersey.
1790s	Local boards of health organized in Baltimore, Boston, Philadelphia, and New York City.
1798	Marine Hospital Service established by Congress. (Now the U.S. Public Health Service.)
1805	First formally organized medical library founded in Boston.
1812	*New England Journal of Medicine* precursor founded. (Now the oldest U.S. medical journal.)
1836	Library of the Surgeon General's Office established, forerunner of the National Library of Medicine.
1842	First use of ether anesthesia by Crawford Long, M.D., in Georgia.
1846	First public demonstration of ether anesthesia at the Massachusetts General Hospital, Boston.
1847	American Medical Association founded.
1851	Female Medical College of Pennsylvania (Philadelphia) founded, world's first medical college for women.

1855	First state health department established in Louisiana.
1861	First voluntary health association, the Civil War Sanitary Commission, founded in New York City.
1872	American Public Health Association formed.
1873	First three U.S. schools of nursing founded, in Boston, New Haven, and New York City.
1879	National Board of Health established, first organized medical research program of the federal government.
1881	American Red Cross founded by Clara Barton.
1887	Charles Mayo, M.D., and his sons established a practice in Rochester, Minnesota, that evolved into the first large medical group practice, the Mayo Clinic.
1891	National Confederation of State Medical Examining and Licensing Boards founded.
1892	Anti-Tuberculosis Society of Philadelphia founded.
1893	Johns Hopkins University School of Medicine founded; offered first formal progressive clinical education of physicians.
1896	X-ray technique used in the United States.
1899	American Hospital Association founded.
1901	Rockefeller Institute for Medical Research founded; first American institute devoted wholly to biomedical research.
	American Medical Association reorganized as a federation of state medical societies.
1902	Parke, Davis & Company (Detroit) began first American, commercially operated research laboratory.
1906	Pure Food and Drug Act passed; became the basis for federal regulation of foods and drugs.
1910	Abraham Flexner's report, "Medical Education in the United States and Canada," published, changing the shape of medical education.
1913	American College of Surgeons founded.
1917	First medical specialty board formed, American Board of Ophthalmology.
1918	First federal grants given to states for public health services.
1929	Blue Cross started at Baylor University (Dallas, Texas).
1930	National Institute of Health (NIH) created. (now called National Institutes of Health)
1935	Social Security Act passed.
1937	Health Service Plan Commission organized. (Later called the Blue Cross Commission.)
	National Cancer Institute of NIH established.
1938	Federal Food, Drug, and Cosmetic Act passed, increasing drug regulation.

1942	First health maintenance organization formed, Kaiser Permanente Health Plan. Rhode Island became first state to enact a health insurance law.
1944	Public Health Service Act passed, extending to all NIH institutes the authority to award research grants to nonfederal agencies.
1946	Hill Burton hospital planning and construction legislation passed to improve population/bed ratios, especially in rural areas.
	Blue Shield Medical Care Plan organized. (Later called the Blue Shield Medical Care Commission.)
1946	Communicable Disease Center established in Atlanta, Georgia. (Now called Centers for Disease Control and prevention.)
1950	National Science Foundation established.
1951	Joint Commission on Accreditation of Hospitals formed. (Now called Joint Commission on Accreditation of Healthcare Organizations.)
1953	Department of Health, Education, and Welfare established as a cabinet level agency. (Now the Department of Health and Human Services.)
1962	Amendments to the Food, Drug, and Cosmetic Act passed, which empowered FDA to specify testing procedures for evaluating new drug applications.
1963	Health Professions Educational Assistance Act legislated to support medical schools and health-related educational institutions.
1964	Nurse Training Act legislated to support nurse training. National Library of Medicine began MEDLARS, the first computerized system for searching medical literature.
1965	Medicare (medical health insurance for citizens over 65) and Medicaid (medical assistance program for the indigent) legislation passed.
	Regional Medical Programs Act passed, establishing regional cooperation in health care planning.
1966	Allied Health Professions Personnel Act legislated to support training of allied health workers.
1968	Health Manpower Act legislated to support training health professionals.
1970	Occupational Safety and Health Act (OSHA) passed, regulating health hazards in the workplace.
	National Institute of Alcohol Abuse and Alcoholism established.
1972	Social Security Act Amendments passed, creating professional service review organizations.

1973	Health Maintenance Organization Act passed, providing funding for model HMO projects.
1974	National Institute on Aging established within NIH.
1975	Rhode Island became first state to enact a catastrophic health insurance program.
1976	Health Care Financing Administration established.
1981	Acquired immunodeficiency syndrome (AIDS) first recognized.
1982	Health Resources and Services Administration established. Orphan Drug Act passed.
	Professional Standards Review Organizations transformed into Peer Review Organizations.
1983	Diagnosis-related groups (DRGs) instituted as method of Medicare reimbursement.
1987	FDA adopted rule allowing release of experimental drugs (e.g., azidothymidine) to individuals with AIDS and other serious diseases.

Source: Data from Joellen Beck Watson Hawkins and Loretta Peirfedeici Higgins, *Nursing and the American Heatlh Care Delivery System* (New York: Tiresias, 1982), 58–60; Theodor J. Litman and Leonard S. Robins, *Health Politics and Policy* (Albany, N.Y.: Delmar, 1991), 395–411; and Florence A. Wilson and Duncan Neuhauser, *Health Services in the United States* (Cambridge, Mass.: Ballinger, 1985), 289–91.

APPENDIX B

Health-Related Discipline History Centers

The following list of repositories collecting manuscripts in various fields within the history of health care is meant to be used to devise cooperative collecting arrangements and to locate appropriate respositories in which to house collections. Institutional archives are not listed.

Anesthesiology

> Wood Library–Museum of Anesthesiology
> 515 Busse Highway
> Park Ridge, IL 60068-3189
> 708/825-5586

Dentistry

> American Dental Association
> Archives
> 211 East Chicago Avenue
> Chicago, IL 60611
> 312/440-2642

> University of Pennsylvania
> School of Dental Medicine
> Library
> 4001 Spruce Street A1
> Philadelphia, PA 19104
> 215/898-8978

Dermatology

> Dermatology Foundation of Miami
> Tape Studio and Library
> 480 Casuarina Concourse
> Coral Gables, FL 33143
> 305/667-3224

Family Medicine

> American Academy of Family Physicians
> 8880 Ward Parkway
> P.O. Box 8418
> Kansas City, MO 64114
> 816/333-9700

Gerontology

> Syracuse University Gerontology Center
> Brockway Hall
> Syracuse, NY 13210
> 315/423-3335

Health—Connecticut, Bridgeport

> Bridgeport Public Library
> Historical Collections
> 925 Broad Street
> Bridgeport, CT 06604
> 203/576-7417

Health Care

> InterStudy
> Library—Information Center
> 5715 Christmas Lake Road
> P.O. Box 458
> Excelsior, MN 55331
> 612/474-1176

> Yale University
> Sterling Memorial Library
> Manuscripts and Archives
> 120 High Street
> Box 1603A Yale Station
> New Haven, CT 06520
> 203/432-1749

Health Care—Alabama

JCMS—UAB Health Sciences Archives
901 18th Street South
Birmingham, AL 35256
205/933-8601

Health Care—Texas

University of Texas Health Science Center at San Antonio
Library—Special Collections
7703 Floyd Curl Drive
San Antonio, TX 78284
512/691-6271

Health Care Administration

Center for Hospital and Health Care Administration History
American Hospital Association
840 North Lake Shore Drive
Chicago, IL 60611
312/280-6258

Health Sciences—California, especially San Francisco

University of California
Library and Center for Knowledge Management
Special Collections and University Archives
San Francisco, CA 94143-0840
415/476-8112

Health Sciences—Michigan

Historical Center for the Health Sciences
715 North University, Suite 6
University of Michigan
Ann Arbor, MI 48104-1611
313/996-9443

History of Medicine—Arkansas

University of Arkansas for Medical Sciences
History of Medicine Division/Archives
Library/Slot 586
Little Rock, AR 72205
501/686-5980

History of Medicine—Connecticut, Hartford

Hartford Medical Society
Library
230 Scarborough Street
Hartford, CT 06105
203/236-5613

History of Medicine—Illinois (Chicago)

University of Illinois at the Medical Center
Library of the Health Sciences
Archives and Special Collections
1750 West Polk Street
P.O. Box 7509
Chicago, IL 60680
312/966-8977

History of Medicine—Los Angeles

University of California—Los Angeles
Biomedical Library
History and Special Collections Division
12-007 Center for the Health Sciences
Los Angeles, CA 90024
213/825-6940

History of Medicine—Maryland

Medical and Chirurgical Faculty of the State of Maryland
Library
1211 Cathedral Street
Baltimore, MD 21201
301/539-0872 x215

History of Medicine—Missouri

St. Louis Metropolitan Medical Society
Oak Knoll Park
Clayton, MO 63105
314/726-2888

History of Medicine—Nebraska

University of Nebraska
Medical Center
Library of Medicine
42nd and Dewey Avenue
Omaha, NE 68105
402/559-7091

History of Medicine—New England, especially Boston

Francis A. Countway Library of Medicine
Special Collections
10 Shattuck Street
Boston, MA 02115
617/732-2171

History of Medicine—New Jersey

University of Medicine and Dentistry of New Jersey
Special Collections and Archives
G. F. Smith Library
30 12th Avenue
Newark, NJ 07103
201/456-6293

History of Medicine—New York

The New York Academy of Medicine Library
Malloch Rare Book and History of Medicine Room
2 East 103rd Street
New York, NY 10029
212/876-8200

New York Hospital—Cornell Medical Center
Medical Archives
1300 York Avenue
New York, NY 10021
212/746-6072

History of Medicine—Ohio (Southwestern)

University of Cincinnati
Libraries
Archives and Rare Book Department
Blegan Library—Room 808
Cincinnati, OH 45221-0113
513/566-1959

History of Medicine—Ohio (Western Reserve)

Cleveland Health Sciences Library
Historical Division
11000 Euclid Avenue
Cleveland, OH 44106
216/368-3648, 3649

History of Medicine—Pennsylvania (esp. Philadelphia) and the U.S.

College of Physicians of Philadelphia
Historical Collections
19 South 22nd Street
Philadelphia, PA 19103
215/561-6050

History of Medicine—Rhode Island

Rhode Island Medical Society
Library
106 Francis Street
Providence, RI 02903
401/331-3208

History of Medicine—South Carolina

Medical University of South Carolina
Health Affairs Library
Waring Historical Library
80 Barre Street
Charleston, SC 29401
803/792-2288

History of Medicine—Texas

Texas Medical Association
Memorial Library
1801 North Lamar Boulevard
Austin, TX 78701
512/477-6704

University of Texas Medical Branch
Moody Medical Library
History of Medicine and Archives Department
Galveston, TX 77550
409/761-2397

History of Medicine—Texas, Harris County and Houston

HAM-TMA Library
Texas Medical Center
1133 M. D. Anderson Boulevard
Houston, TX 77030
713/797-1230 x139

History of Medicine—United States

American Philosophical Society
Library
105 South 5th Street
Philadelphia, PA 19106
215/440-3409

National Library of Medicine
History of Medicine Division
Bethesda, MD 20894
301/496-5963

Smithsonian Institution
National Museum of American History
Department of History of Science and Technology
Division of Medical Sciences
AHB 5000
12th Street and Constitution Avenue, N.W.
Washington, DC 20560
202/357-3270

University of Kansas Medical Center
College of Health Sciences and Hospital
Clendening History of Medicine Library
Rainbow Boulevard at 39th Street
Kansas City, KS 66103
913/588-7040

History of Medicine—Wisconsin

Medical College of Wisconsin
Todd Wehr Library
8701 Watertown Plank Road
P.O. Box 26509
Milwaukee, WI 53226
414/257-8302

Hospitals

Center for Hospitals and Health Care Administration History
American Hospital Association
840 North Lake Shore Drive
Chicago, IL 60611
312/280-6258

Internal Medicine

American College of Physicians
Archives
4200 Pine Street
Philadelphia, PA
215/243-1200

Microbiology

Center for the History of Microbiology
Albin O. Kuhn Library and Gallery
University of Maryland–Baltimore County
Baltimore, MD 21228
301/455-3601

Military Medicine

Armed Forces Institute of Pathology
Armed Forces Medical Museum
Otis Historical Archives
Alaska Avenue and 14th Street, N.W.
Washington, DC 20306
202/576-2334, 2341, 2348

Neurology

Archives of Neurology
American Association of Neurological Surgeons
22 South Washington Street
Park Ridge, IL 60068
708/629-9500

Nursing

Nursing History Archives
Mugar Library
Boston University
771 Commonwealth Avenue
Boston, MA 02215
617/353-3696

Center for the Study of the History of Nursing
University of Pennsylvania
Nursing Education Building/S2
Philadelphia, PA 19104
215/898-4502

Oncology Nursing Society
501 Holiday Drive
Pittsburgh, PA 15220-2749
412/921-7373

Nutrition

Vanderbilt University
Medical Center Library
Special Collections
Nashville, TN 37232
615/322-0008

Obstetrics and Gynecology

American College of Obstetrics and Gynecology
Historical Collection
409 Twelfth Street, S.W.
Washington, DC 20024
202/638-5577

Ophthalmology

Foundation of the American Academy of Ophthalmology
Department of Ophthalmic Heritage
655 Beach Street
P.O. Box 6988
San Francisco, CA 94101-6988
415/561-8500

Otolaryngology

American Academy of Otolaryngology—Head and
Neck Surgery
Department of Archives and History
1 Prince Street
Alexandria, VA 22314
703/836-4444

Pediatrics

American Academy of Pediatrics
141 Northwest Point Boulevard
Elk Grove Village, IL 60009
708/981-4722

Pharmacy

American Institute of the History of Pharmacy
Pharmacy Building
University of Wisconsin
Madison, WI 53706
608/262-2894

University of Pennsylvania
Van Pelt Library
Edgar Fahs Smith Collection in the History of Chemistry
3420 Walnut Street
Philadelphia, PA 19104
212/898-7088

Physical Therapy and Rehabilitation

Abbott–Northwestern Hospital Corporation
Sister Kenny Institute
800 East 28th Street
Minneapolis, MN 55407
612/874-4312

Plastic Surgery

Columbia University Health Sciences Library
Special Collections
701 West 168th Street
New York, NY 10032
212/305-7931

Psychiatry

American Psychiatric Association Archives
1400 "K" Street, N.W.
Washington, DC 20005
202/682-6017

Public Health

University of Minnesota
Libraries
Social Welfare History Archives
101 Walter Library
117 Pleasant Street, S.E.
Minneapolis, MN 55445
612/624-6394

Women in Medicine

Medical College of Pennsylvania
Archives and Special Collections on Women in Medicine
3300 Henry Avenue
Philadelphia, PA 19129
215/842-7124

Radcliffe College
Arthur and Elizabeth Schlesinger Library on the History of Women in America
10 Garden Street
Cambridge, MA 02138
617/495-8647, 8648

INDEX